INCLUDES ADVICE AND PROMPTS FOR EVERY SKIN TYPE!

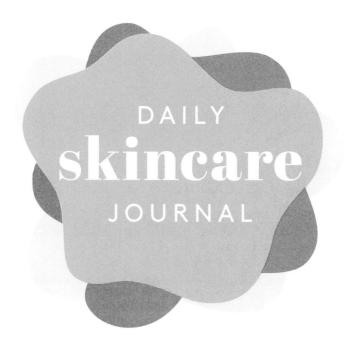

DAILY
skincare
JOURNAL

From Testing New Products to
Tracking Your Daily Routine,
Your Guide to the Best Skin Ever!

MARIA DEL RUSSO

ADAMS MEDIA
NEW YORK   LONDON   TORONTO   SYDNEY   NEW DELHI

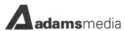

Adams Media
An Imprint of Simon & Schuster, Inc.
100 Technology Center Drive
Stoughton, Massachusetts 02072

First Adams Media hardcover edition March 2023

ADAMS MEDIA and colophon are trademarks of Simon & Schuster.

For information about special discounts for bulk purchases, please contact Simon & Schuster Special Sales at 1-866-506-1949 or business@simonandschuster.com.

The Simon & Schuster Speakers Bureau can bring authors to your live event. For more information or to book an event contact the Simon & Schuster Speakers Bureau at 1-866-248-3049 or visit our website at www.simonspeakers.com.

Interior design by Colleen Cunningham
Interior images © blankstock; 123RF/zubada

Manufactured in the United States of America

1 2022

ISBN 978-1-5072-2025-2

Contents

Introduction   5

How to Use This Book   7

PART 1: **A Beginner's Guide to Skin Care** 10
Chapter 1: Allow Us to Introduce You to...Your Skin 12

PART 2: **Establishing Your Skincare Routine** 28
My Skin Assessment 30
My Skincare Goals 31
My Favorite Products Tracker 32
New Products I'm Trying Tracker 34
Expiration Tracker 37

PART 3: **Your Morning and Nighttime Routine Trackers** . . . 40

APPENDIX: Additional Resources 222

ACKNOWLEDGMENTS

To all of my beauty industry friends and former editors, thank you for your love, lessons, and all of the inspiration you bring to our world. And to everyone who has ever emailed, DM'd, tweeted, or texted me a skincare question...here! I wrote this for you.

Introduction

"How do I improve my skin?"

It's the number one question any dermatologist, beauty writer, or skincare guru hears. And with good reason! Your face is the first thing you present to the world. However, it's not always easy to figure out *how* to get the skin you want. There are so many skincare trends out there—from abrasions, to creams, to masks—it can get a bit confusing and overwhelming. Fortunately, *Daily Skincare Journal* will help you pinpoint the specific needs of your skin and find the best solutions to any problems you may be having.

No matter your age, gender, or skin tone, the secret to your best skin ever is simple: consistency. Finding the right products for your skin takes a little bit of trial and error. But once you do, the most important step you can take toward clearer skin is returning to those products day after day. The more you're able to find a routine and stick to it, the easier it will be to get the results you've always desired. That's why the trackers in this book are so important. With them, you will have a record of what products worked (or didn't work), your skincare goals and how they are progressing, and even those pesky expiration dates. You can track your routine every day, morning and night, so that you can fall into a daily skincare routine that's simple to maintain.

In the following pages, you'll get a crash course in skin care. You'll find information on identifying your skin type, figuring out how to find the right products for you, learning how to layer products, and how to know when products expire. You'll also be provided with a handy guide to some of those trickier skincare phrases, how certain medications affect your face, and when it's time to talk to a dermatologist.

Speaking of a dermatologist, it's a good idea to talk to yours before you kick off any major skincare overhaul. Don't have a derm? Your primary care doctor is a pretty good alternative. If price or distance is an issue, it's super easy to "see" a dermatologist via telehealth. The Appendix of this book can help you with a handful of good options for app-based dermatologists.

This journal is meant to help you become more comfortable with your regimen and the skin you've got. Because, in truth, the best skin is the one that protects your inside from the outside. A clearer, more glowing complexion? That's just the cherry on top.

So gather your cleansers, toners, and serums. It's time to dive in!

How to Use This Book

No matter where you are in your skincare journey, this book can help guide you. Starting completely from scratch? This book has you covered. Finding that your typical routine doesn't have the same oomph it used to? This journal can still be incredibly useful. Your skin care needs to evolve and change as you age. Your skin can also grow accustomed to a routine if you've been using it for a while. So if your results are stalling, it could just mean you need to change things up a bit, whether that means swapping in a new cleanser or introducing an entirely new product into your routine.

The first part of this book is your guide to skin care. Although it's tailored to those who are just starting out in the skincare game, it's a great refresher for everyone—and a resource you can refer back to as you progress through the rest of this journal. In this guide, you'll learn how to identify your skin type, the correct order in which to layer products, and how to keep track of your products' expiration dates. (Yes, they do expire, and you don't want them on your skin once they do!)

You'll also get a quick breakdown of the most common skincare phrases and tips on how to know when to call your dermatologist. Not every skin concern can be cured at home with over-the-counter products. Sometimes it's a good idea to call the pros to bring in the big guns.

Once you've learned all the basics, you can start tracking. *Daily Skincare Journal* has two types of trackers for you to use: lists you fill out once and those you'll fill out over time. These trackers will help you identify your skincare goals, new products you're testing, and when those products expire. They start out with a skincare assessment, so you can take a clear look at your major skincare concerns and figure out the right steps forward. In the assessment, you'll identify what your goals are for your skincare routine. Do you want to reduce breakouts? Treat your discoloration? That's important to identify so you can track your progress. You'll also be asked to fill out information on how your skin makes you feel. There are also trackers for listing out your favorite products so you can keep track as you're testing, as well as for evaluating new products you're trying with star ratings.

The most important parts of this book, however, are the daily skincare trackers. They give you the space to track your morning and evening routines over the course of three months down to the precise details. Why three months? It's a common belief that it takes a little over two months to form a habit. But it also takes about three months for you to start to notice any significant change in your skin after adopting a new routine. You can list off the products you use (so you never again forget whether you used your retinol last night) and take notes of things like stress, where you're breaking out, any tools you may use, and how much water you drink in a day. There's also a section called Other Notes, where you can track any medication you take to control breakouts, how much sleep you got the night before, what foods you've been eating that you think are affecting your skin, where you are in your menstrual cycle (if applicable), or anything else you feel is important. This may be the most important part of the trackers because it's a place where you can note any changes in your skin, specifically how it's evolving over time. You can even use this section to track any treatments you've received from your dermatologist and how your skin is reacting to them.

Here's the thing, though—there isn't a right way to use this book. You're not going to get a gold star if you fill out each section perfectly every day. You may find some of the trackers are more useful than others. You may not have any medications to keep an eye on. The most important part is that you keep with it, no matter how much you fill out in a day.

Consistency is the key to healthy skin, and the trackers in this book try to make it as simple as possible to maintain that consistency. Try keeping this journal in your bathroom or your bedside table—anywhere where it will be easy to remember to fill it out every day. Over time, you'll be able to identify patterns in your routine and how your skin is reacting, which should make it easier to figure out triggers and flares for different skincare issues.

And remember, this journal doesn't have to be used in any particular order once you get started. So don't be afraid to hop around! As long as you are consistently filling out your daily routine trackers, you'll eventually fall into a routine that is so seamless it will become second nature.

PART 1

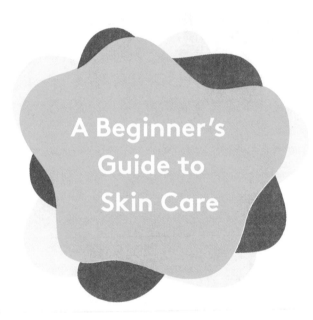

A Beginner's
Guide to
Skin Care

If you're new to the idea of building a skincare routine, you're probably wondering what all the fuss is about. Everyone has skin, so why does it seem like there are a billion different ways of caring for it? The answer is simple—not all skin types are the same. There is a range of factors that affect the care and keeping of your dermis, from your age to your skin color, even the weather where you live. With all of these factors that go into skincare maintenance, is it any wonder that there is a nearly $100 billion market dedicated to skin?

Before you start treating your skin, it's a good idea to get familiar with it first. Like a lot of your biology, skin type is largely dictated by your genetics, which is why you and your siblings may have similar skin issues. And even though there isn't an "acne gene," a researcher named Hugo Hecht found in the 1960s that breakouts do run in families. (So make sure to thank your parents the next time you're dealing with a breakout ahead of a big meeting!)

Unfortunately, it can feel super overwhelming to get started on a skincare routine. Just walking down the beauty aisles of your local drugstore can be enough to make your head spin. So before you begin tracking your routines, it's important to learn the basics of skin care.

Keep reading for your beginner's guide to understanding your skin. It's a lot of information up front, but once you have it under your belt, you'll be well on your way to conquering your skincare woes.

Allow Us to Introduce You to...Your Skin

As you can probably imagine, identifying your skin tone and type are the first steps in figuring out how to care for your skin. This chapter will break down the characteristics of each skin type and give you tips on how to identify the way your skin behaves. Once your skin type is defined, this chapter will help you build a routine from scratch—or just help fill in the blanks where you need them.

You'll also learn about how to choose the right products for your skin type, including active ingredients to treat everything from dryness to shine, as well as the different types of breakouts and how to treat each one. You'll learn the correct way to layer products, tips for applying different types of products, a rundown of common skincare phrases, and how to know when your bottles and tubes have expired. Still stumped? This chapter will walk you through when it's a good idea to contact your dermatologist.

Consider the following info your crash course in skin care. And remember that this chapter is always available for you to refer back to as you work your way through your routine. Remember to check back whenever you're feeling a little lost.

Identifying Your Skin Tone

Skin tone is essentially the color of your skin. Melanin is the pigment that gives your skin its color, and the more melanin you have, the darker your skin tone is. You've probably also heard of the term "undertone." That refers to the subtle hue beneath your skin tone, which is the top layer. Melanin actually acts as a protector against the sun, so those with deeper skin tones are less likely to suffer from sunburns, freckles, skin cancer, and other ailments that come from the sun. But melanin alone isn't enough to protect you from ultraviolet rays, so it's still important to wear sunblock, no matter how dark your skin is.

Those with higher melanin content may also be susceptible to other skin conditions, such as hyperpigmentation, flesh moles, and dry skin. Hyperpigmentation is a big issue for these skin tones, especially regarding procedures such as chemical peels and lasers, as well as skin-brightening products, like vitamin C. It's especially important for those with deeper skin tones to chat with a doctor or a dermatologist before trying anything that may cause hyperpigmentation. When in doubt, test on a small patch of your skin for a few weeks and see how your skin reacts. If you have any change in skin tone or any other adverse reaction, stop using that product immediately and give your doctor a call.

Skin tones tend to fall into three main categories: light, medium, and dark. Especially when discussing makeup, there tends to be a bunch of subcategories under these three main categories. This book doesn't go into those subcategories because they are unregulated and differ from brand to brand. But your main skin tone should be easy to identify just by looking in the mirror!

- **Light skin tones** indicate the least amount of melanin in the skin. People with this skin tone tend to burn easily and have a lot of freckles. These people are typically from Northern Europe.
- **Medium skin tones** are found among people who come from Southern Europe and North Asia. They tend to tan very easily but can still sunburn. This skin tone is sometimes called "olive."
- **Dark skin tones** indicate the most amount of melanin in the skin. Those with this skin tone come from places with the highest exposure to UV (ultraviolet) rays, like the Middle East,

Africa, and India. Although they don't tend to burn, they can still suffer from sun damage, so it's important that those with deeper skin tones still wear sunscreen.

Identifying Your Skin Type

While skin tone is about the color of your skin, "skin type" refers to how your skin behaves. According to the American Academy of Dermatology, there are five skin types, each with its own unique characteristics:

- **Dry skin** feels tight, itchy, or rough throughout the day. You may experience flakiness, peeling, or a dull tone to your face, especially when you're in colder temperatures. Dry skin is caused by an underproduction of sebum, aka your skin's natural oil. (Yes, some oil is actually good for your skin!)
- **Oily skin** has the opposite problem—it overproduces sebum, which makes your face look greasy or shiny. You may also notice other skin concerns like blackheads or enlarged pores. Every skin type experiences breakouts, but oily types are more prone to pimples, since those enlarged pores are more easily clogged with excess sebum.
- **Sensitive skin** can appear red or inflamed after coming into contact with stressors, including certain skincare products. Your skin may itch, tingle, or burn after using a product. If you deal with other skin conditions, like rosacea or eczema, there is a good chance your skin is sensitive.
- **Combination skin** is, you guessed it, a *combination* of at least two of the previous skin types. A lot of people with combination skin have an oily T-zone (your forehead, nose, and chin) but dry cheeks. That's not the standard, though. Combination skin just means your skin has different characteristics on different parts of your face.

- **Normal skin** is the term used to describe skin that doesn't display any of the previous characteristics, including acne. That said, *all* skin is normal, regardless of how it is defined, so don't let this term get you down!

If you're not sure which category you fall into, there's an easy way to find out. Wash your face with a gentle cleanser (that means *no* active ingredients) and then pat it dry with a towel. Don't apply any more skincare products. Instead, wait about a half hour and then see how your skin looks and feels. Is your face super greasy? You probably have oily skin. Are just your cheeks dry? You may be classified as having combination skin. Does it feel rough or tight? Your skin may be on the drier side. If your skin is irritated or red, that points to sensitivity.

It's important to note that your skin will change as you get older, which means you may have to redefine your skin type. Aging skin is thinner, thanks to a loss of collagen and fat, so it may be more sensitive. But those with older skin also may experience dryness because people tend to lose sweat and oil glands as they age. It's a good idea to do the preceding test every few years or when your skincare routine doesn't seem to be as effective. You may need totally new products!

Choosing the Right Products for Your Skin Type

Now that you've got your skin type down, it's important to know how to treat it. Each skin type has its own unique set of needs, as well as products and ingredients that can further exacerbate any problems or symptoms. So when shopping for skincare products, here are some things to keep in mind for your skin type:

Dry Skin

If you have dry skin, stick with a gentle moisturizing cleanser in cream or gel form, since foaming cleansers can further strip your skin of natural oils. For moisturizers, reach for creams over gels or lotions.

In the winter, it's a good idea to lock in your moisturizer with a face oil at the end of your routine. Oils will create a protective barrier over your skin, holding in place whatever moisturizing products you've put on your face. Look for ingredients like glycerin, ceramides, and hyaluronic acid. These are humectants, which help your skin retain its moisture.

You want to avoid anything drying, like alcohols, benzoyl peroxide, and salicylic acid. Artificial fragrances can also sap your skin of moisture, so try to stay away from those too.

Oily Skin

Cleansing is an important step for oily skin types, so be sure to find products with active ingredients like salicylic acid or glycolic acid. Retinols can help keep your breakouts at bay, but it's important to check in with your dermatologist before starting one, as it can take your skin time to adjust, and they aren't right for everyone. (Pregnant women, for example, shouldn't use retinol.) When you moisturize, skip the gloopy creams and choose a lightweight lotion or gel.

Stay away from heavier products, as they can be comedogenic, which means they can clog pores. Petroleum jelly and cocoa butter are the main ingredients to steer clear of, but you also want to skip oils. Your skin produces plenty already!

Combination Skin

This can be the trickiest skin type to treat, since your face needs different things all over. It's a good idea to stick with gentle cleansers without any harsh ingredients and then use your treatment products (like retinol or hyaluronic acid) where you need them most. Gel moisturizers tend to be the best for all-over use with combination skin, as they provide plenty of hydration without clogging pores.

Make sure to avoid harsh ingredients on your dry areas and anything oil-based on your oily areas. It's also a good idea to avoid alcohol and preservatives like parabens, since they can exacerbate *both* oily and dry skin—and that's the exact opposite of what you want.

Sensitive Skin

The most important thing for sensitive skin types to remember is this: "Gentle" is the name of the game. Opt for cleansers with very few ingredients. Most dermatologists will recommend a cleanser like Cetaphil or CeraVe for sensitive skin types, as they're as bare bones as you can get. You should also look for moisturizers that are formulated specifically for sensitive skin, as they will be free of any ingredients that will inflame your tender dermis.

Make sure to keep your routine clear of anything active, like benzoyl peroxide, salicylic acid, or retinols. Fragrances and alcohol can also cause irritation or stinging, so stay away from those too.

Normal Skin

If you don't fall into any of these categories, there isn't a whole lot that will irritate your skin (lucky you!). That said, if you notice any breakouts, dryness, or irritation when using a new product, it's a good idea to discontinue using it. In general, though, a simple routine of a gentle cleanser, a moisturizer, and a sunscreen should be perfectly fine for you, although you may need to adjust depending on the time of year or the weather.

Breakout Types and How to Treat Them

If you were to go by the movies, the only type of breakout anyone ever gets is a huge red bump with a big white dot in the center of it. But if you deal with breakouts, you probably know this isn't the case. "Acne" is actually an umbrella term for any and every bump that crops up when your pores or hair follicles become clogged with oil and dead skin. But there are different types of breakouts, and knowing which kind you have is important so that you can properly treat it. Here's how to know what you're working against.

Blackheads and Whiteheads

While they may look super different, blackheads and whiteheads are actually both caused by clogged pores due to excess oil, dead skin, or bacteria. They are sometimes slightly raised from the skin and can feel hard. The only difference? If the skin grows over the top of the pore, you'll see a white or skin-colored bump. That's a whitehead. Blackheads occur when the skin *doesn't* grow over the pore. Instead, the oil and dirt inside the pore oxidize to create a little black speck that might look like a dot of pepper.

The best way to treat blackheads and whiteheads is to unclog the pores with active ingredients. Retinols are great at reducing the number of blackheads and whiteheads. It's also a good idea to look for a face wash with benzoyl peroxide, which penetrates pores and kills acne-causing bacteria. It's important not to pick whiteheads or blackheads because doing so can cause scarring.

Papules

This is where things tend to get confusing. Papules are a type of pimple, but not the ones you think of when you hear the word "zit." These are small, red, inflamed breakouts that are hard and can be painful. But they don't have any head to them, meaning there isn't any pus visible. These are really common among people going through puberty, and it's normal to have clusters of them on your forehead or chin. Papules can also be treated with benzoyl peroxide. Salicylic acid is another great ingredient for this type of acne. It's a BHA, or a beta hydroxy acid, which exfoliates the skin and helps to unclog your pores. It's also an anti-inflammatory, so it will help shrink your pimples in size over time.

Pustule

Ah, pustules. These are your classic pimples—red, angry-looking zits that look similar to papules. But unlike papules, which look the same all over, pustules have a yellowish or white dot of pus on top.

The most important thing to know about pustules is that you should not pick them. Yes, it can be tempting, but picking and squeezing these zits can inflame them further, which can delay the natural healing process. It can also spread bacteria, making you break out more. But what's worse, picking pustules can actually cause permanent scarring. Instead, use a benzoyl peroxide or salicylic acid wash or treatment. If your pustules are really bad, it's a good idea to chat with a dermatologist.

Cysts and Nodules

Cysts and nodules are caused by bacteria, dead skin, or oil that burrows deep into the skin. These breakouts tend to be large, inflamed, and *really* tender. They are the most severe form of acne and usually appear in large clusters on the face. Cysts contain pus and may have a white head. But nodules are solid and hard because they don't contain fluid. These can be super painful to the touch, but like with pustules, whiteheads, and blackheads, it's important not to pick them. Cysts and nodules are the breakouts most likely to scar, so they need to be treated with care.

These types of breakouts are notoriously difficult to treat with over-the-counter ingredients. If you have this type of acne, it's important to schedule an appointment with a dermatologist. The treatment of cysts and nodules usually includes some type of prescription topical or an oral antibiotic. But although nodules are painful, it's important to know that they are almost always treatable with the help of an expert. So don't let them get you down!

Do My Skincare Products Expire?

Like most things, skincare products have a shelf life that is important to keep an eye on. If you use a product that has expired, it can cause all sorts of issues, from a little tingling sensation to serious skin issues or chemical burns. That's because a lot of skincare products use active ingredients, and they only stay stable for a certain amount of time.

Every skincare product should have an indicator on its package that lets you know its shelf life once opened. This is called the "period after opening" symbol. It looks like a little open jar and usually has a number with the letter "M" next to it. The M stands for "months," so 6M means six months from opening, 12M means a year, and so on. But if a product has a funky smell or a change in color, or if it appears to be separating, thickening, or thinning, it may mean it's gone bad, so it's a good idea to toss it. Most products will stay good between a year to two years, with natural ingredients degrading more quickly than synthetic ones.

The Correct Way to Layer Skincare Products

Believe it or not, there is a right way and a wrong way to apply your products to your skin to ensure the active ingredients are able to penetrate your dermis correctly. To achieve maximum efficacy, you should order your products like this:

1. Cleanser
2. Toner
3. Eye Cream
4. Serum
5. Retinol or Other Treatments (p.m. only)
6. Spot Treatment
7. Moisturizer
8. Sunscreen (a.m. only)

If you're using multiple products that fit into one of these categories, or if you get stumped on the order in which you should apply, remember the golden rule of skin care: Always go with the product with the thinnest consistency first and work your way up to your thickest consistency.

How Do I Apply My Products?

To get the most benefit out of your skincare products, it's important to apply them in the correct way. The biggest mistake people make when applying their products is that they move too quickly and apply too much pressure. In general, you want to use a lighter touch when applying your products. The skin on your face is delicate and should be treated gently! Here's a breakdown of how to apply your products:

- **Cleanser:** Using your fingers, massage your face with big, circular, upward motions. Make sure to get around the sides of your nose—you can use smaller up-and-down motions here.
- **Face Scrub:** You want to make circular motions like with your cleanser, but they should be smaller. Make sure to avoid the sensitive skin around your eyes!
- **Toner:** You can apply toner either by sprinkling a bit onto a cotton pad and sweeping it over your skin or by dropping a bit onto your fingertips and pressing it into your skin. It's really up to personal preference.
- **Eye Cream:** The skin around your eyes is *very* delicate, so tap in your eye cream. Some say that your ring finger is best, since it naturally applies the least amount of pressure, but as long as you tap lightly, it doesn't matter which finger you use!
- **Serum:** Unlike a moisturizer, you want to pat a serum into your skin instead of rubbing it in. Patting with your fingertips allows it to absorb the way it's formulated to, so avoid the temptation to rub it in.
- **Oils:** These are one of the only products that is applied with your entire hand—not just the fingers or fingertips. Rub a small amount over your hand and then gently pat the oil into the skin.
- **Moisturizer:** You can be a little firmer with your moisturizer just to ensure proper absorption. Apply it with your fingertips in an outward motion.

A Quick Breakdown of Skincare Phrases

Skin care can be *super* confusing. It can sometimes feel like you need a PhD in chemistry just to choose a cleanser! But all it takes is a little research. Following, you'll find a handful of common words and phrases used in the beauty industry and their definitions. This is by no means an exhaustive list, but there are plenty of resources online if you ever get confused. (You can also find a list of them in the back of this book!)

Accutane

Accutane is a powerful medication that is used to treat super severe cystic acne. It's only available by prescription from your dermatologist, and it's usually reserved for when your acne hasn't responded to other treatments.

Alpha Hydroxy Acids (AHAs)

You're most likely to see AHAs in acne-fighting products and anti-aging creams. That's because this acid is a powerful exfoliant. AHAs work to break down the bonds between dead skin cells, which means they get washed away, leaving newer skin cells to shine. Glycolic acid is a type of AHA, and you'll typically find it in peels and cleansers.

Antioxidants

"Antioxidant" is an umbrella term for any ingredient that protects the skin against free radicals. Free radicals are the unstable molecules your body produces when you're exposed to things like pollution, smoke, or sunlight. These molecules damage your skin cells, leading them to break down, which can cause your skin to appear rough or wrinkled. Antioxidants work to prevent that damage.

Beta Hydroxy Acids (BHAs)

Like AHAs, BHAs are a chemical exfoliant. But there's one major difference. While AHAs work to remove dead skin cells from the *surface* of the skin, BHAs penetrate deeply into pores, helping to excavate dead skin and oil buildup. (An easy way to remember the difference is that AHAs start with "A" and work "above" the skin, while BHAs start with "B" and work "below" the skin.) Salicylic acid is a type of BHA, and you'll typically see it in acne-fighting products.

Broad Spectrum

When a sunscreen is listed as "broad spectrum," it means it defends against both UVA (ultraviolet A, which is associated with skin aging) and UVB (ultraviolet B, associated with skin burning) rays. The Food and Drug Administration (FDA) suggests wearing broad-spectrum sunscreens with an SPF of at least 15 and reapplying regularly.

Ceramides

This term refers to something that is both an ingredient *and* a naturally occurring part of your skin. Ceramides are the fatty acids that keep the cells of your skin together and keep the skin barrier strong. But synthetic ceramides also exist in skin care and work just like the ones that naturally occur in your skin. (In fact, they tend to be more stable!) Since they actually work to heal the epidermis, you'll typically find them in moisturizers for people with really dry or sensitive skin types.

Collagen

Your skin is about 80 percent collagen. Collagen is a protein that helps the skin stay firm and strong, but, like most things, it breaks down as you age. There are different ways to regain collagen, however. Dermatologists offer both laser treatments and injectables that can help rebuild lost collagen volume. At home, a good retinoid regimen can help stimulate your skin to produce new collagen naturally.

Doxycycline

Known as "doxy" for short, this is another prescribed medication for acne. It's actually an antibiotic, so it kills acne-causing bacteria and works to lower inflammation. Doxycycline is usually only pre-scribed as a short-term solution because if it is used for too long, the bacteria can become resistant to the treatment.

Eczema

Eczema is a skin disorder that causes scaly, itchy patches of skin. These patches are usually red and can be made worse by scratching. Those with eczema are usually also classified as having sensitive skin, as harsh soaps and fragrances can make their rashes worse. You usually see eczema in children, although adults can be diagnosed too, and it usually pops up on or around the elbows, knees, eyes, or neck.

Hyperpigmentation

This condition is characterized as a darkening of the skin, whether by the sun, hormonal changes (like pregnancy), or other factors. When your skin tans after being out in the sun, that's hyper-pigmentation! It may also appear as melasma, which is when your skin develops dark patches, or as a scar after you injure your skin.

Melanin

This is the technical name for the pigment that gives your skin its color. (Melanin also colors your hair and eyes, FYI.) The darker your skin is, the higher the melanin content.

Melanoma

An uncommon, but very serious, form of skin cancer. It usually presents as a mole that changes in size, shape, color, or feel. Mela-noma is the most serious type of skin cancer because it can spread. But according to the Skin Cancer Foundation, when melanoma is detected early, the five-year survival rate is 99 percent. It's important to get your moles checked regularly by a dermatologist, especially if you spend a lot of time out in the sun, so melanoma can be detected early if it develops. You can and should regularly perform a self-check at home. You can check out the Skin Cancer Foundation's website for a step-by-step guide to self-exams.

Parabens

You've probably heard that parabens are bad. Parabens are a preservative that helps to keep bacteria and fungi from growing in your products. Studies have shown that they can disrupt hormones in the body, which may lead to an increased risk of cancers, fertility issues, and other problems. But there's been no conclusive answer as to whether they are truly bad for you, and the FDA says they're safe in small amounts—like less than half a percent—in cosmetics.

Pores

These are the small openings in your skin that allow oil and sweat to escape. Pores are present all over the skin, but there is a higher concentration of them on your face. No matter what a product says it can do, pores cannot open or close. They cannot shrink or be erased. Pores look larger when they are clogged, but using products like AHAs, BHAs, and sunscreen can help reduce their appearance.

Retinoids

This is the umbrella term for all derivatives of vitamin A that are used in skincare products. Retinol is the most commonly known form of vitamin A. Retin-A is a brand name for prescription tretinoin, which is a more concentrated form of vitamin A than retinol.

Rosacea

Like eczema, rosacea is a chronic skin disease, but this one is characterized by redness on the nose and cheeks more than itching. People with rosacea tend to flush easily and are susceptible to more broken blood vessels and pimples. Rosacea also tends to run in families, so if your parents have it, there's a good chance you do too. Those with rosacea should treat their skin as sensitive.

Sebum

Although it gets a bad rep, sebum is actually produced by your skin's sebaceous glands to protect it. It's an oily, waxy substance made up of fatty acids, sugars, and other natural chemicals. The terms "sebum" and "oil" are used interchangeably when referring to acne, but zit-causing oils are actually more complex. They contain sebum but also sweat and other buildup on your skin that react and create breakouts.

Skin Barrier

Your skin barrier refers to the outermost layer of your skin, known as the stratum corneum. Think of it like a brick wall that defends the more delicate layers of skin beneath it from the elements. It consists of two main parts: skin cells, known as "corneocytes," and lipids, which are fatty acids and ceramides that hold them together. A strong skin barrier is important to healthy skin.

SPF

Sun protection factor (SPF) is a fancy way of saying "how long sunscreen will protect you from UV rays." So if your sunscreen has an SPF of 20, you'll be protected twenty times longer than if you had not worn sunscreen. That said, reapplication every two hours or after swimming is recommended, no matter the SPF level, because SPF wears off more quickly when exposed to the elements.

Spironolactone

Spironolactone is another acne-fighting medication that you can only get with a prescription. It's a diuretic that protects potassium, which is why its main use is to lower blood pressure. Its acne-fighting power comes from its ability to block testosterone, which can cause hormonal acne in certain people. Since it isn't an antibiotic, it can be used for long periods. That's why it's useful for people who have chronic hormonal acne. An antibiotic like doxycycline, however, is more useful for those with more topical causes of zits.

When to Call a Dermatologist

While the information in this journal is a good starting place, it's important to have regular appointments with your dermatologist. Checking in with your doctor will not only keep the skin on your face healthy; it will also help you keep tabs on the rest of your body. Regular skin checks are the easiest and most effective way to catch skin cancers before they develop. Dermatologists will also help guide you when introducing new products into your routine, especially if you're using something with super strong active ingredients.

In general, these are the times when you should look to a dermatologist's expertise—not the Internet:

- You notice a mole or patch of skin that is new or looks different than you remember whether because of its size, shape, color, or symptom.
- You have really stubborn acne that isn't responding to over-the-counter treatments.
- You're experiencing a new rash or itch that you haven't before.
- You experience a tingling or burning sensation when using a new product. (You should also stop using that product immediately—skin care should never hurt!)
- You have a scrape or other lesion that won't heal.
- Your skin is red all the time, no matter what you use on it.

If you notice any of these issues, make an appointment with your doctor. Make sure to note any new products you've been using or treatments you've been trying. Luckily, the skincare trackers in this journal have an Other Notes section just for that!

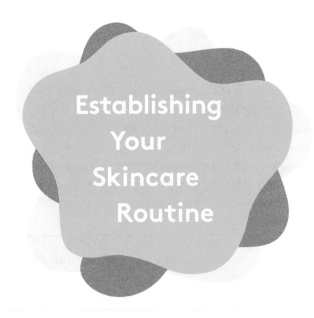

PART 2

Establishing
Your
Skincare
Routine

Now that you've gotten to know your skin a little bit better, you're ready to start building your routine from scratch. There's a good chance you already have a handful of products that you love to use, whether it's a foaming cleanser that keeps your acne at bay or a hyaluronic acid gel cream that hydrates your skin without feeling too heavy. That's a great starting point! There's no need to toss out your favorites and start from zero. Instead, you can figure out your needs by first assessing what you want to achieve in your skincare journey.

The following part has a handful of templates for you to fill out that will help identify your starting point. You'll start by taking a good look at your skin in the My Skin Assessment template. Here, you'll identify trouble areas and how you hope to heal them. But you'll also think about how your skin makes you feel, since a lot of how you're feeling on the inside can actually show up on your epidermis. Once you establish where you are today, you can figure out where you want to go tomorrow. You'll be asked to think about your skincare goals and how you hope to achieve them. As with most habits in life, having a specific goal will keep you on track so that you're more likely to stick to your routine day after day.

And those products you are already loving? There's a place for you to list them out, as well as space for you to jot down any new favorites you discover through your skincare journey. You'll also be able to track new products you're testing and give them a review, as well as keep an eye on when your products expire with the Expiration Tracker. All of these templates are designed to help keep you on track and think of your skincare routine in a full 360-degree way. So let's get started!

my skin assessment

My skin type:

My skin tone:

How my skin makes me feel:

Where my skincare concerns are:

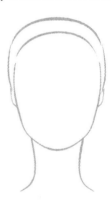

My current skincare regimen:

Medications/treatments I use:

my skincare goals

MY MAIN SKINCARE CONCERN(S):

○ Acne   ○   ○
○ Uneven skin tone   ○   ○
○ Fine lines/wrinkles   ○   ○
○ Dark spots   ○   ○
○ Lack of glow   ○   ○

FOCUS:

Changes I want to make:

How I want my skin to make me feel:

My biggest skincare hurdle:

Where I want my skin to be in ninety days:

my favorite products tracker

☐ CLEANSER:

☐ TONER:

☐ SERUMS:

☐ SPOT TREATMENTS:

☐ EYE CREAM:

☐ MOISTURIZER:

☐ FACE OIL:

☐ SUNSCREEN:

☐ RETINOL:

☐ EXFOLIANT:

☐ FACE MASKS:

CLEANSER:

TONER:

SERUMS:

SPOT TREATMENTS:

EYE CREAM:

MOISTURIZER:

FACE OIL:

SUNSCREEN:

RETINOL:

EXFOLIANT:

FACE MASKS:

new products i'm trying tracker

☐ _____ ★ ★ ★ ★ ★

☐ _____ ★ ★ ★ ★ ★

☐ _____ ★ ★ ★ ★ ★

☐ _____ ★ ★ ★ ★ ★

☐ _____ ★ ★ ★ ★ ★

☐ _____ ★ ★ ★ ★ ★

☐ _____ ★ ★ ★ ★ ★

☐ _____ ★ ★ ★ ★ ★

☐ _____ ★ ★ ★ ★ ★

☐ _____ ★ ★ ★ ★ ★

☐ _____ ★ ★ ★ ★ ★

✔ PRODUCT NAME	START DATE	STAR RATING

new products i'm trying tracker

☐   ☆ ☆ ☆ ☆ ☆

☐   ☆ ☆ ☆ ☆ ☆

☐   ☆ ☆ ☆ ☆ ☆

☐   ☆ ☆ ☆ ☆ ☆

☐   ☆ ☆ ☆ ☆ ☆

☐   ☆ ☆ ☆ ☆ ☆

☐   ☆ ☆ ☆ ☆ ☆

☐   ☆ ☆ ☆ ☆ ☆

☐   ☆ ☆ ☆ ☆ ☆

☐   ☆ ☆ ☆ ☆ ☆

☐   ☆ ☆ ☆ ☆ ☆

expiration tracker

✔	PRODUCT NAME	DATE OPENED	PERIOD AFTER OPENING DATE
☐			
☐			
☐			
☐			
☐			
☐			
☐			
☐			
☐			
☐			
☐			
☐			

expiration tracker

✔	PRODUCT NAME	DATE OPENED	PERIOD AFTER OPENING DATE
☐			
☐			
☐			
☐			
☐			
☐			
☐			
☐			
☐			
☐			
☐			
☐			

✔	PRODUCT NAME	DATE OPENED	PERIOD AFTER OPENING DATE
☐			
☐			
☐			
☐			
☐			
☐			
☐			
☐			
☐			
☐			
☐			
☐			

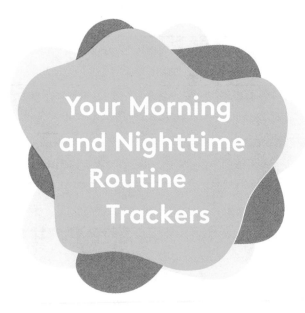

PART 3

Your Morning and Nighttime Routine Trackers

Congratulations! You've gotten your crash course in the basics of skin care, identified your goals, and started listing off products you're loving and the ones you plan to test. Now is the fun part: getting into your skincare routine.

The following templates should be used twice a day: once in the morning and once in the evening. In these templates, you'll be able to check off your products as you go to ensure you're never missing a step. But as this book has established, skin care is more than what you put on your face. These templates allow you to take a holistic approach to your dermis. You'll have the opportunity to write down how your skin is feeling and how you yourself are feeling, because both of those things can have an effect on how your face is behaving that day. You'll also be able to track treatments and tools you're using and how much water you drank that day. There is even a section to note where you're breaking out on your skin so you can track the life cycle of your acne and figure out how your zits are healing.

The most important section, though, may be the Other Notes section. This is where you'll jot down anything else you think may be affecting your skincare journey. It's a good place to note where you are in your menstrual cycle if you have one, any medications you're taking to treat your skin, or any foods you've eaten that may impact how your skin is feeling that day. It's also a good place to note any changes to your skin so that you can tell your dermatologist exactly when those changes began.

The key to using these templates is consistency, so try keeping this journal in a place you know you'll use it twice daily, whether that's in your bedroom, in your bathroom, or at your desk. Once you get through the ninety days, you should see a difference in your skin and be well on your way to maintaining a routine. So good luck, and let's get tracking!

routine tracker

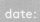

MORNING ROUTINE

TODAY MY SKIN FEELS:

TODAY I FEEL:

OTHER NOTES:

SKINCARE STEPS:

- ○ Cleanser
- ○ Toner
- ○ Spot Treatment
- ○ Serums
    - ○
    - ○
    - ○
- ○ Eye Cream
- ○ Moisturizer
- ○ Face Oil
- ○ Sunscreen
    - ○
    - ○
    - ○

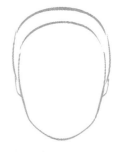

where I'm breaking out

EXTRA STEPS:

- ○ Exfoliation
- ○ Face Mask
- ○ Face Massage
- ○
- ○

TOOLS I USED:

- ○ Gua Sha
- ○ Microcurrent Device
- ○ Jade Roller
- ○ Ice Roller
- ○

| 8oz | 8oz | 8oz | 8oz |
| 8oz | 8oz | 8oz | 8oz |

WATER INTAKE

EVENING ROUTINE

TONIGHT MY SKIN FEELS:

TONIGHT I FEEL:

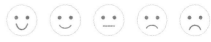

OTHER NOTES:

SKINCARE STEPS:

- ○ Cleanser
- ○ Toner
- ○ Spot Treatment
- ○ Serums
  - ○
  - ○
  - ○

- ○ Eye Cream
- ○ Moisturizer
- ○ Face Oil
- ○
- ○
- ○
- ○

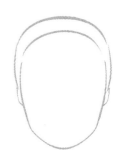

where I'm breaking out

EXTRA STEPS:

- ○ Exfoliation
- ○ Retinol
- ○ Face Mask
- ○
- ○

- ○
- ○
- ○
- ○
- ○

OTHER NOTES:

routine tracker

MORNING ROUTINE

TODAY MY SKIN FEELS:

TODAY I FEEL:

OTHER NOTES:

SKINCARE STEPS:

- ○ Cleanser
- ○ Toner
- ○ Spot Treatment
- ○ Serums
  - ○
  - ○
  - ○

- ○ Eye Cream
- ○ Moisturizer
- ○ Face Oil
- ○ Sunscreen
  - ○
  - ○
  - ○

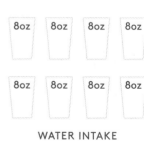

where I'm breaking out

EXTRA STEPS:

- ○ Exfoliation
- ○ Face Mask
- ○ Face Massage
- ○
- ○

TOOLS I USED:

- ○ Gua Sha
- ○ Microcurrent Device
- ○ Jade Roller
- ○ Ice Roller
- ○

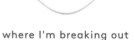

| 8oz | 8oz | 8oz | 8oz |
| 8oz | 8oz | 8oz | 8oz |

WATER INTAKE

44

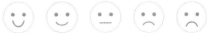

EVENING ROUTINE

TONIGHT MY SKIN FEELS:

TONIGHT I FEEL:

OTHER NOTES:

SKINCARE STEPS:

○ Cleanser ○ Eye Cream
○ Toner ○ Moisturizer
○ Spot Treatment ○ Face Oil
○ Serums ○
  ○ ○
  ○ ○
  ○ ○

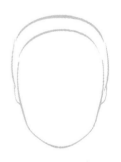

where I'm breaking out

EXTRA STEPS:

OTHER NOTES:

○ Exfoliation ○
○ Retinol ○
○ Face Mask ○
○ ○
○ ○

routine tracker

MORNING ROUTINE

TODAY MY SKIN FEELS:

TODAY I FEEL:

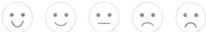

OTHER NOTES:

SKINCARE STEPS:

- ○ Cleanser
- ○ Toner
- ○ Spot Treatment
- ○ Serums
  - ○
  - ○
  - ○

- ○ Eye Cream
- ○ Moisturizer
- ○ Face Oil
- ○ Sunscreen
  - ○
  - ○
  - ○

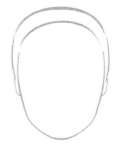

where I'm breaking out

EXTRA STEPS:

- ○ Exfoliation
- ○ Face Mask
- ○ Face Massage
- ○
- ○

TOOLS I USED:

- ○ Gua Sha
- ○ Microcurrent Device
- ○ Jade Roller
- ○ Ice Roller
- ○

8oz	8oz	8oz	8oz
8oz	8oz	8oz	8oz

WATER INTAKE

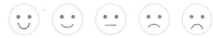
EVENING ROUTINE

TONIGHT MY SKIN FEELS:

TONIGHT I FEEL:

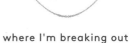

OTHER NOTES:

SKINCARE STEPS:

- ○ Cleanser
- ○ Toner
- ○ Spot Treatment
- ○ Serums
- ○
- ○
- ○

- ○ Eye Cream
- ○ Moisturizer
- ○ Face Oil
- ○
- ○
- ○
- ○

where I'm breaking out

EXTRA STEPS:

- ○ Exfoliation
- ○ Retinol
- ○ Face Mask
- ○
- ○

- ○
- ○
- ○
- ○
- ○

OTHER NOTES:

routine tracker

MORNING ROUTINE

TODAY MY SKIN FEELS:

TODAY I FEEL:

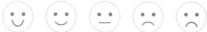

OTHER NOTES:

SKINCARE STEPS:

- ○ Cleanser
- ○ Toner
- ○ Spot Treatment
- ○ Serums
  - ○
  - ○
  - ○

- ○ Eye Cream
- ○ Moisturizer
- ○ Face Oil
- ○ Sunscreen
  - ○
  - ○
  - ○

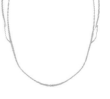

where I'm breaking out

EXTRA STEPS:

- ○ Exfoliation
- ○ Face Mask
- ○ Face Massage
- ○
- ○

TOOLS I USED:

- ○ Gua Sha
- ○ Microcurrent Device
- ○ Jade Roller
- ○ Ice Roller
- ○

| 8oz | 8oz | 8oz | 8oz |
| 8oz | 8oz | 8oz | 8oz |

WATER INTAKE

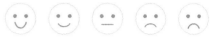

weather: sleep:

EVENING ROUTINE

TONIGHT MY SKIN FEELS:

TONIGHT I FEEL:

OTHER NOTES:

SKINCARE STEPS:

○ Cleanser
○ Toner
○ Spot Treatment
○ Serums
  ○
  ○
  ○

○ Eye Cream
○ Moisturizer
○ Face Oil
○
○
○
○

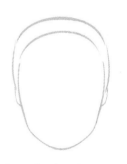

where I'm breaking out

EXTRA STEPS:

○ Exfoliation
○ Retinol
○ Face Mask
○
○

○
○
○
○
○

OTHER NOTES:

49

routine tracker

MORNING ROUTINE

TODAY MY SKIN FEELS:

TODAY I FEEL:

OTHER NOTES:

SKINCARE STEPS:

- ○ Cleanser
- ○ Toner
- ○ Spot Treatment
- ○ Serums
  - ○
  - ○
  - ○
- ○ Eye Cream
- ○ Moisturizer
- ○ Face Oil
- ○ Sunscreen
  - ○
  - ○
  - ○

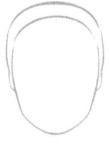

where I'm breaking out

EXTRA STEPS:

- ○ Exfoliation
- ○ Face Mask
- ○ Face Massage
- ○
- ○

TOOLS I USED:

- ○ Gua Sha
- ○ Microcurrent Device
- ○ Jade Roller
- ○ Ice Roller
- ○

| 8oz | 8oz | 8oz | 8oz |
| 8oz | 8oz | 8oz | 8oz |

WATER INTAKE

EVENING ROUTINE

TONIGHT MY SKIN FEELS:

TONIGHT I FEEL:

OTHER NOTES:

SKINCARE STEPS:

- ○ Cleanser
- ○ Toner
- ○ Spot Treatment
- ○ Serums
  - ○
  - ○
  - ○

- ○ Eye Cream
- ○ Moisturizer
- ○ Face Oil
- ○
- ○
- ○
- ○

where I'm breaking out

OTHER NOTES:

EXTRA STEPS:

- ○ Exfoliation
- ○ Retinol
- ○ Face Mask
- ○
- ○

- ○
- ○
- ○
- ○
- ○

routine tracker

MORNING ROUTINE

TODAY MY SKIN FEELS:

TODAY I FEEL:

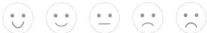

OTHER NOTES:

SKINCARE STEPS:

- ○ Cleanser
- ○ Toner
- ○ Spot Treatment
- ○ Serums
  - ○
  - ○
  - ○

- ○ Eye Cream
- ○ Moisturizer
- ○ Face Oil
- ○ Sunscreen
  - ○
  - ○
  - ○

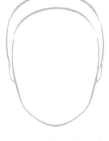

where I'm breaking out

EXTRA STEPS:

- ○ Exfoliation
- ○ Face Mask
- ○ Face Massage
- ○
- ○

TOOLS I USED:

- ○ Gua Sha
- ○ Microcurrent Device
- ○ Jade Roller
- ○ Ice Roller
- ○

| 8oz | 8oz | 8oz | 8oz |
| 8oz | 8oz | 8oz | 8oz |

WATER INTAKE

EVENING ROUTINE

TONIGHT MY SKIN FEELS:

TONIGHT I FEEL:

OTHER NOTES:

SKINCARE STEPS:

○ Cleanser   ○ Eye Cream

○ Toner   ○ Moisturizer

○ Spot Treatment   ○ Face Oil

○ Serums   ○

　○   ○

　○   ○

　○   ○

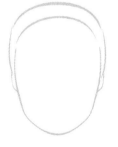

where I'm breaking out

EXTRA STEPS: OTHER NOTES:

○ Exfoliation   ○

○ Retinol   ○

○ Face Mask   ○

○   ○

○   ○

routine tracker

MORNING ROUTINE

TODAY MY SKIN FEELS:

TODAY I FEEL:

OTHER NOTES:

SKINCARE STEPS:

- ○ Cleanser
- ○ Toner
- ○ Spot Treatment
- ○ Serums
  - ○
  - ○
  - ○

- ○ Eye Cream
- ○ Moisturizer
- ○ Face Oil
- ○ Sunscreen
  - ○
  - ○
  - ○

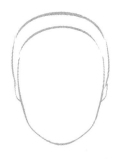

where I'm breaking out

EXTRA STEPS:

- ○ Exfoliation
- ○ Face Mask
- ○ Face Massage
- ○
- ○

TOOLS I USED:

- ○ Gua Sha
- ○ Microcurrent Device
- ○ Jade Roller
- ○ Ice Roller
- ○

8oz	8oz	8oz	8oz
8oz	8oz	8oz	8oz

WATER INTAKE

EVENING ROUTINE

TONIGHT MY SKIN FEELS:

TONIGHT I FEEL:

    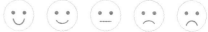

OTHER NOTES:

SKINCARE STEPS:

- ○ Cleanser
- ○ Toner
- ○ Spot Treatment
- ○ Serums
  - ○
  - ○
  - ○

- ○ Eye Cream
- ○ Moisturizer
- ○ Face Oil
- ○
- ○
- ○
- ○

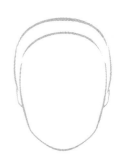

where I'm breaking out

EXTRA STEPS:

OTHER NOTES:

- ○ Exfoliation
- ○ Retinol
- ○ Face Mask
- ○
- ○

- ○
- ○
- ○
- ○
- ○

routine tracker

MORNING ROUTINE

TODAY MY SKIN FEELS:

TODAY I FEEL:

OTHER NOTES:

SKINCARE STEPS:

- ○ Cleanser
- ○ Toner
- ○ Spot Treatment
- ○ Serums
    - ○
    - ○
    - ○

- ○ Eye Cream
- ○ Moisturizer
- ○ Face Oil
- ○ Sunscreen
    - ○
    - ○
    - ○

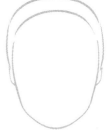

where I'm breaking out

EXTRA STEPS:

- ○ Exfoliation
- ○ Face Mask
- ○ Face Massage
- ○
- ○

TOOLS I USED:

- ○ Gua Sha
- ○ Microcurrent Device
- ○ Jade Roller
- ○ Ice Roller
- ○

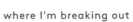

| 8oz | 8oz | 8oz | 8oz |
| 8oz | 8oz | 8oz | 8oz |

WATER INTAKE

EVENING ROUTINE

TONIGHT MY SKIN FEELS:

TONIGHT I FEEL:

OTHER NOTES:

SKINCARE STEPS:

○ Cleanser   ○ Eye Cream
○ Toner   ○ Moisturizer
○ Spot Treatment   ○ Face Oil
○ Serums   ○
   ○   ○
   ○   ○
   ○   ○

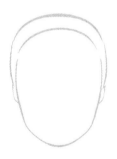

where I'm breaking out

EXTRA STEPS:

OTHER NOTES:

○ Exfoliation   ○
○ Retinol   ○
○ Face Mask   ○
○   ○
○   ○

routine tracker

MORNING ROUTINE

TODAY MY SKIN FEELS:

TODAY I FEEL:

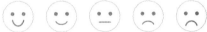

OTHER NOTES:

SKINCARE STEPS:

- ○ Cleanser
- ○ Toner
- ○ Spot Treatment
- ○ Serums
    - ○
    - ○
    - ○

- ○ Eye Cream
- ○ Moisturizer
- ○ Face Oil
- ○ Sunscreen
    - ○
    - ○
    - ○

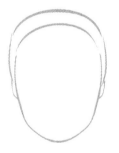

where I'm breaking out

EXTRA STEPS:

- ○ Exfoliation
- ○ Face Mask
- ○ Face Massage
- ○
- ○

TOOLS I USED:

- ○ Gua Sha
- ○ Microcurrent Device
- ○ Jade Roller
- ○ Ice Roller
- ○

8oz	8oz	8oz	8oz
8oz	8oz	8oz	8oz

WATER INTAKE

EVENING ROUTINE

TONIGHT MY SKIN FEELS:

TONIGHT I FEEL:

OTHER NOTES:

SKINCARE STEPS:

- ○ Cleanser
- ○ Toner
- ○ Spot Treatment
- ○ Serums
  - ○
  - ○
  - ○

- ○ Eye Cream
- ○ Moisturizer
- ○ Face Oil
- ○
- ○
- ○
- ○

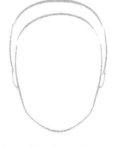

where I'm breaking out

EXTRA STEPS:

- ○ Exfoliation
- ○ Retinol
- ○ Face Mask
- ○
- ○

- ○
- ○
- ○
- ○
- ○

OTHER NOTES:

routine tracker

MORNING ROUTINE

TODAY MY SKIN FEELS:

TODAY I FEEL:

OTHER NOTES:

SKINCARE STEPS:

- ○ Cleanser
- ○ Toner
- ○ Spot Treatment
- ○ Serums
    - ○
    - ○
    - ○
- ○ Eye Cream
- ○ Moisturizer
- ○ Face Oil
- ○ Sunscreen
    - ○
    - ○
    - ○

where I'm breaking out

EXTRA STEPS:

- ○ Exfoliation
- ○ Face Mask
- ○ Face Massage
- ○
- ○

TOOLS I USED:

- ○ Gua Sha
- ○ Microcurrent Device
- ○ Jade Roller
- ○ Ice Roller
- ○

| 8oz | 8oz | 8oz | 8oz |
| 8oz | 8oz | 8oz | 8oz |

WATER INTAKE

EVENING ROUTINE

TONIGHT MY SKIN FEELS:

TONIGHT I FEEL:

 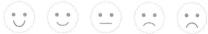

OTHER NOTES:

SKINCARE STEPS:

○ Cleanser ○ Eye Cream
○ Toner ○ Moisturizer
○ Spot Treatment ○ Face Oil
○ Serums ○
　○ ○
　○ ○
　○ ○

where I'm breaking out

EXTRA STEPS:

OTHER NOTES:

○ Exfoliation ○
○ Retinol ○
○ Face Mask ○
○ ○
○ ○

routine tracker

MORNING ROUTINE

TODAY MY SKIN FEELS:

TODAY I FEEL:

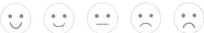

OTHER NOTES:

SKINCARE STEPS:

- ○ Cleanser
- ○ Toner
- ○ Spot Treatment
- ○ Serums
    - ○
    - ○
    - ○

- ○ Eye Cream
- ○ Moisturizer
- ○ Face Oil
- ○ Sunscreen
    - ○
    - ○
    - ○

where I'm breaking out

EXTRA STEPS:

- ○ Exfoliation
- ○ Face Mask
- ○ Face Massage
- ○
- ○

TOOLS I USED:

- ○ Gua Sha
- ○ Microcurrent Device
- ○ Jade Roller
- ○ Ice Roller
- ○

8oz	8oz	8oz	8oz
8oz	8oz	8oz	8oz

WATER INTAKE

EVENING ROUTINE

TONIGHT MY SKIN FEELS:

TONIGHT I FEEL:

  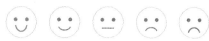

OTHER NOTES:

SKINCARE STEPS:

- ○ Cleanser
- ○ Toner
- ○ Spot Treatment
- ○ Serums
  - ○
  - ○
  - ○

- ○ Eye Cream
- ○ Moisturizer
- ○ Face Oil
- ○
- ○
- ○
- ○

where I'm breaking out

EXTRA STEPS:

- ○ Exfoliation
- ○ Retinol
- ○ Face Mask
- ○
- ○

- ○
- ○
- ○
- ○
- ○

OTHER NOTES:

routine tracker

 date:

MORNING ROUTINE

TODAY MY SKIN FEELS:

TODAY I FEEL:

  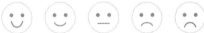

OTHER NOTES:

SKINCARE STEPS:

○ Cleanser   ○ Eye Cream
○ Toner   ○ Moisturizer
○ Spot Treatment   ○ Face Oil
○ Serums   ○ Sunscreen
  ○   ○
  ○   ○
  ○   ○

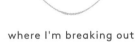

where I'm breaking out

EXTRA STEPS:

○ Exfoliation
○ Face Mask
○ Face Massage
○
○

TOOLS I USED:

○ Gua Sha
○ Microcurrent Device
○ Jade Roller
○ Ice Roller
○

| 8oz | 8oz | 8oz | 8oz |
| 8oz | 8oz | 8oz | 8oz |

WATER INTAKE

EVENING ROUTINE

TONIGHT MY SKIN FEELS:

TONIGHT I FEEL:

OTHER NOTES:

SKINCARE STEPS:

- ○ Cleanser
- ○ Toner
- ○ Spot Treatment
- ○ Serums
  - ○
  - ○
  - ○

- ○ Eye Cream
- ○ Moisturizer
- ○ Face Oil
- ○
- ○
- ○
- ○

where I'm breaking out

EXTRA STEPS:

- ○ Exfoliation
- ○ Retinol
- ○ Face Mask
- ○
- ○

- ○
- ○
- ○
- ○
- ○

OTHER NOTES:

routine tracker

MORNING ROUTINE

TODAY MY SKIN FEELS:

TODAY I FEEL:

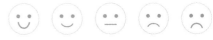

OTHER NOTES:

SKINCARE STEPS:

- ○ Cleanser
- ○ Toner
- ○ Spot Treatment
- ○ Serums
- ○
- ○
- ○

- ○ Eye Cream
- ○ Moisturizer
- ○ Face Oil
- ○ Sunscreen
- ○
- ○
- ○

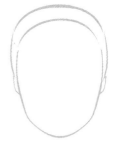

where I'm breaking out

EXTRA STEPS:

- ○ Exfoliation
- ○ Face Mask
- ○ Face Massage
- ○
- ○

TOOLS I USED:

- ○ Gua Sha
- ○ Microcurrent Device
- ○ Jade Roller
- ○ Ice Roller
- ○

8oz	8oz	8oz	8oz

8oz	8oz	8oz	8oz

WATER INTAKE

EVENING ROUTINE

TONIGHT MY SKIN FEELS:

TONIGHT I FEEL:

OTHER NOTES:

SKINCARE STEPS:

- O Cleanser
- O Toner
- O Spot Treatment
- O Serums
  - O
  - O
  - O

- O Eye Cream
- O Moisturizer
- O Face Oil
- O
- O
- O
- O

where I'm breaking out

EXTRA STEPS:

- O Exfoliation
- O Retinol
- O Face Mask
- O
- O

- O
- O
- O
- O
- O

OTHER NOTES:

routine tracker

MORNING ROUTINE

TODAY MY SKIN FEELS:

TODAY I FEEL:

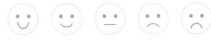

OTHER NOTES:

SKINCARE STEPS:

- ○ Cleanser
- ○ Toner
- ○ Spot Treatment
- ○ Serums
  - ○
  - ○
  - ○

- ○ Eye Cream
- ○ Moisturizer
- ○ Face Oil
- ○ Sunscreen
  - ○
  - ○
  - ○

where I'm breaking out

EXTRA STEPS:

- ○ Exfoliation
- ○ Face Mask
- ○ Face Massage
- ○
- ○

TOOLS I USED:

- ○ Gua Sha
- ○ Microcurrent Device
- ○ Jade Roller
- ○ Ice Roller
- ○

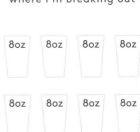

WATER INTAKE

EVENING ROUTINE

TONIGHT MY SKIN FEELS:

TONIGHT I FEEL:

OTHER NOTES:

SKINCARE STEPS:

○ Cleanser   ○ Eye Cream

○ Toner   ○ Moisturizer

○ Spot Treatment   ○ Face Oil

○ Serums   ○

    ○   ○

    ○   ○

    ○   ○

where I'm breaking out

EXTRA STEPS:

OTHER NOTES:

○ Exfoliation   ○

○ Retinol   ○

○ Face Mask   ○

○   ○

○   ○

routine tracker

MORNING ROUTINE

TODAY MY SKIN FEELS:

TODAY I FEEL:

OTHER NOTES:

SKINCARE STEPS:

- Cleanser
- Toner
- Spot Treatment
- Serums
  - ○
  - ○
  - ○

- Eye Cream
- Moisturizer
- Face Oil
- Sunscreen
  - ○
  - ○
  - ○

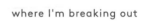

where I'm breaking out

EXTRA STEPS:

- Exfoliation
- Face Mask
- Face Massage
- ○
- ○

TOOLS I USED:

- Gua Sha
- Microcurrent Device
- Jade Roller
- Ice Roller
- ○

| 8oz | 8oz | 8oz | 8oz |
| 8oz | 8oz | 8oz | 8oz |

WATER INTAKE

EVENING ROUTINE

TONIGHT MY SKIN FEELS:

TONIGHT I FEEL:

OTHER NOTES:

SKINCARE STEPS:

○ Cleanser   ○ Eye Cream
○ Toner   ○ Moisturizer
○ Spot Treatment   ○ Face Oil
○ Serums   ○
  ○   ○
  ○   ○
  ○   ○

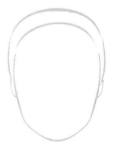

where I'm breaking out

EXTRA STEPS: **OTHER NOTES:**

○ Exfoliation   ○
○ Retinol   ○
○ Face Mask   ○
○   ○
○   ○

routine tracker

MORNING ROUTINE

TODAY MY SKIN FEELS:

TODAY I FEEL:

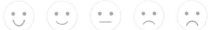

OTHER NOTES:

SKINCARE STEPS:

- ○ Cleanser
- ○ Toner
- ○ Spot Treatment
- ○ Serums
- ○
- ○
- ○

- ○ Eye Cream
- ○ Moisturizer
- ○ Face Oil
- ○ Sunscreen
- ○
- ○
- ○

where I'm breaking out

EXTRA STEPS:

- ○ Exfoliation
- ○ Face Mask
- ○ Face Massage
- ○
- ○

TOOLS I USED:

- ○ Gua Sha
- ○ Microcurrent Device
- ○ Jade Roller
- ○ Ice Roller
- ○

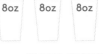

| 8oz | 8oz | 8oz | 8oz |
| 8oz | 8oz | 8oz | 8oz |

WATER INTAKE

EVENING ROUTINE

TONIGHT MY SKIN FEELS:

TONIGHT I FEEL:

OTHER NOTES:

SKINCARE STEPS:

○ Cleanser   ○ Eye Cream

○ Toner   ○ Moisturizer

○ Spot Treatment   ○ Face Oil

○ Serums   ○

  ○   ○

  ○   ○

  ○   ○

where I'm breaking out

EXTRA STEPS:

OTHER NOTES:

○ Exfoliation   ○

○ Retinol   ○

○ Face Mask   ○

○   ○

○   ○

routine tracker

MORNING ROUTINE

TODAY MY SKIN FEELS:

TODAY I FEEL:

OTHER NOTES:

SKINCARE STEPS:

- ○ Cleanser
- ○ Toner
- ○ Spot Treatment
- ○ Serums
- ○ _____
- ○ _____
- ○ _____

- ○ Eye Cream
- ○ Moisturizer
- ○ Face Oil
- ○ Sunscreen
- ○ _____
- ○ _____
- ○ _____

where I'm breaking out

EXTRA STEPS:

- ○ Exfoliation
- ○ Face Mask
- ○ Face Massage
- ○ _____
- ○ _____

TOOLS I USED:

- ○ Gua Sha
- ○ Microcurrent Device
- ○ Jade Roller
- ○ Ice Roller
- ○ _____

8oz	8oz	8oz	8oz
8oz	8oz	8oz	8oz

WATER INTAKE

74

EVENING ROUTINE

TONIGHT MY SKIN FEELS:

TONIGHT I FEEL:

OTHER NOTES:

SKINCARE STEPS:

- ○ Cleanser
- ○ Toner
- ○ Spot Treatment
- ○ Serums
    - ○
    - ○
    - ○

- ○ Eye Cream
- ○ Moisturizer
- ○ Face Oil
- ○
- ○
- ○
- ○

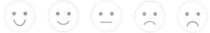

where I'm breaking out

EXTRA STEPS:

- ○ Exfoliation
- ○ Retinol
- ○ Face Mask
- ○
- ○

- ○
- ○
- ○
- ○
- ○

OTHER NOTES:

routine tracker

MORNING ROUTINE

TODAY MY SKIN FEELS:

TODAY I FEEL:

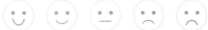

OTHER NOTES:

SKINCARE STEPS:

- ◯ Cleanser
- ◯ Toner
- ◯ Spot Treatment
- ◯ Serums
  - ◯
  - ◯
  - ◯

- ◯ Eye Cream
- ◯ Moisturizer
- ◯ Face Oil
- ◯ Sunscreen
  - ◯
  - ◯
  - ◯

where I'm breaking out

EXTRA STEPS:

- ◯ Exfoliation
- ◯ Face Mask
- ◯ Face Massage
- ◯
- ◯

TOOLS I USED:

- ◯ Gua Sha
- ◯ Microcurrent Device
- ◯ Jade Roller
- ◯ Ice Roller
- ◯

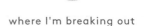

| 8oz | 8oz | 8oz | 8oz |
| 8oz | 8oz | 8oz | 8oz |

WATER INTAKE

EVENING ROUTINE

TONIGHT MY SKIN FEELS:

TONIGHT I FEEL:

OTHER NOTES:

SKINCARE STEPS:

○ Cleanser   ○ Eye Cream
○ Toner   ○ Moisturizer
○ Spot Treatment   ○ Face Oil
○ Serums   ○
   ○   ○
   ○   ○
   ○   ○

where I'm breaking out

EXTRA STEPS: OTHER NOTES:

○ Exfoliation   ○
○ Retinol   ○
○ Face Mask   ○
○   ○
○   ○

routine tracker

MORNING ROUTINE

TODAY MY SKIN FEELS:

TODAY I FEEL:

    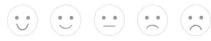

OTHER NOTES:

SKINCARE STEPS:

- ○ Cleanser
- ○ Toner
- ○ Spot Treatment
- ○ Serums
  - ○
  - ○
  - ○

- ○ Eye Cream
- ○ Moisturizer
- ○ Face Oil
- ○ Sunscreen
  - ○
  - ○
  - ○

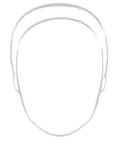

where I'm breaking out

EXTRA STEPS:

- ○ Exfoliation
- ○ Face Mask
- ○ Face Massage
- ○
- ○

TOOLS I USED:

- ○ Gua Sha
- ○ Microcurrent Device
- ○ Jade Roller
- ○ Ice Roller
- ○

| 8oz | 8oz | 8oz | 8oz |
| 8oz | 8oz | 8oz | 8oz |

WATER INTAKE

EVENING ROUTINE

TONIGHT MY SKIN FEELS:

TONIGHT I FEEL:

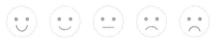

OTHER NOTES:

SKINCARE STEPS:

○ Cleanser   ○ Eye Cream
○ Toner   ○ Moisturizer
○ Spot Treatment ○ Face Oil
○ Serums   ○
    ○   ○
    ○   ○
    ○   ○

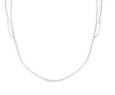

where I'm breaking out

EXTRA STEPS:

○ Exfoliation   ○
○ Retinol   ○
○ Face Mask   ○
○   ○
○   ○

OTHER NOTES:

routine tracker

 date:

MORNING ROUTINE

TODAY MY SKIN FEELS:

TODAY I FEEL:

OTHER NOTES:

SKINCARE STEPS:

○ Cleanser   ○ Eye Cream
○ Toner   ○ Moisturizer
○ Spot Treatment   ○ Face Oil
○ Serums   ○ Sunscreen
   ○   ○
   ○   ○
   ○   ○

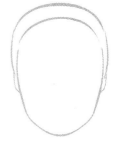

where I'm breaking out

EXTRA STEPS: TOOLS I USED:

○ Exfoliation   ○ Gua Sha
○ Face Mask   ○ Microcurrent Device
○ Face Massage   ○ Jade Roller
○   ○ Ice Roller
○   ○

8oz | 8oz | 8oz | 8oz

8oz | 8oz | 8oz | 8oz

WATER INTAKE

EVENING ROUTINE

TONIGHT MY SKIN FEELS:

TONIGHT I FEEL:

OTHER NOTES:

SKINCARE STEPS:

- ○ Cleanser
- ○ Toner
- ○ Spot Treatment
- ○ Serums
    - ○
    - ○
    - ○

- ○ Eye Cream
- ○ Moisturizer
- ○ Face Oil
- ○
- ○
- ○
- ○

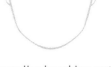

where I'm breaking out

EXTRA STEPS:

- ○ Exfoliation
- ○ Retinol
- ○ Face Mask
- ○
- ○

- ○
- ○
- ○
- ○
- ○

OTHER NOTES:

routine tracker

MORNING ROUTINE

TODAY MY SKIN FEELS:

TODAY I FEEL:

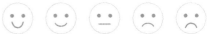

OTHER NOTES:

SKINCARE STEPS:

- ○ Cleanser
- ○ Toner
- ○ Spot Treatment
- ○ Serums
  - ○
  - ○
  - ○

- ○ Eye Cream
- ○ Moisturizer
- ○ Face Oil
- ○ Sunscreen
  - ○
  - ○
  - ○

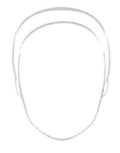

where I'm breaking out

EXTRA STEPS:

- ○ Exfoliation
- ○ Face Mask
- ○ Face Massage
- ○
- ○

TOOLS I USED:

- ○ Gua Sha
- ○ Microcurrent Device
- ○ Jade Roller
- ○ Ice Roller
- ○

8oz	8oz	8oz	8oz
8oz	8oz	8oz	8oz

WATER INTAKE

EVENING ROUTINE

TONIGHT MY SKIN FEELS:

TONIGHT I FEEL:

OTHER NOTES:

SKINCARE STEPS:

- ○ Cleanser
- ○ Toner
- ○ Spot Treatment
- ○ Serums
  - ○
  - ○
  - ○

- ○ Eye Cream
- ○ Moisturizer
- ○ Face Oil
- ○
- ○
- ○
- ○

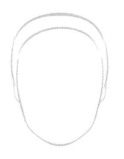

where I'm breaking out

EXTRA STEPS:

- ○ Exfoliation
- ○ Retinol
- ○ Face Mask
- ○
- ○

- ○
- ○
- ○
- ○
- ○

OTHER NOTES:

routine tracker

 date:

MORNING ROUTINE

TODAY MY SKIN FEELS: TODAY I FEEL:

OTHER NOTES:

SKINCARE STEPS:

○ Cleanser   ○ Eye Cream
○ Toner   ○ Moisturizer
○ Spot Treatment   ○ Face Oil
○ Serums   ○ Sunscreen
   ○   ○
   ○   ○
   ○   ○

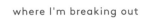

where I'm breaking out

EXTRA STEPS: TOOLS I USED:

○ Exfoliation   ○ Gua Sha
○ Face Mask   ○ Microcurrent Device
○ Face Massage   ○ Jade Roller
○   ○ Ice Roller
○   ○

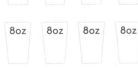

| 8oz | 8oz | 8oz | 8oz |
| 8oz | 8oz | 8oz | 8oz |

WATER INTAKE

EVENING ROUTINE

TONIGHT MY SKIN FEELS:

TONIGHT I FEEL:

OTHER NOTES:

SKINCARE STEPS:

- ○ Cleanser
- ○ Toner
- ○ Spot Treatment
- ○ Serums
  - ○
  - ○
  - ○

- ○ Eye Cream
- ○ Moisturizer
- ○ Face Oil
- ○
- ○
- ○
- ○

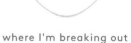

where I'm breaking out

EXTRA STEPS:

- ○ Exfoliation
- ○ Retinol
- ○ Face Mask
- ○
- ○

- ○
- ○
- ○
- ○
- ○

OTHER NOTES:

routine tracker

MORNING ROUTINE

TODAY MY SKIN FEELS:

TODAY I FEEL:

OTHER NOTES:

SKINCARE STEPS:

- ○ Cleanser
- ○ Toner
- ○ Spot Treatment
- ○ Serums
  - ○
  - ○
  - ○

- ○ Eye Cream
- ○ Moisturizer
- ○ Face Oil
- ○ Sunscreen
  - ○
  - ○
  - ○

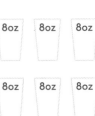

where I'm breaking out

EXTRA STEPS:

- ○ Exfoliation
- ○ Face Mask
- ○ Face Massage
- ○
- ○

TOOLS I USED:

- ○ Gua Sha
- ○ Microcurrent Device
- ○ Jade Roller
- ○ Ice Roller
- ○

| 8oz | 8oz | 8oz | 8oz |
| 8oz | 8oz | 8oz | 8oz |

WATER INTAKE

EVENING ROUTINE

TONIGHT MY SKIN FEELS:

TONIGHT I FEEL:

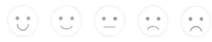

OTHER NOTES:

SKINCARE STEPS:

○ Cleanser   ○ Eye Cream
○ Toner   ○ Moisturizer
○ Spot Treatment ○ Face Oil
○ Serums   ○
   ○   ○
   ○   ○
   ○   ○

where I'm breaking out

EXTRA STEPS: OTHER NOTES:

○ Exfoliation   ○
○ Retinol   ○
○ Face Mask   ○
○   ○
○   ○

routine tracker

MORNING ROUTINE

TODAY MY SKIN FEELS:

TODAY I FEEL:

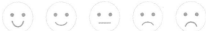

OTHER NOTES:

SKINCARE STEPS:

- ○ Cleanser
- ○ Toner
- ○ Spot Treatment
- ○ Serums
  - ○
  - ○
  - ○ _____

- ○ Eye Cream
- ○ Moisturizer
- ○ Face Oil
- ○ Sunscreen
  - ○
  - ○
  - ○ _____

where I'm breaking out

EXTRA STEPS:

- ○ Exfoliation
- ○ Face Mask
- ○ Face Massage
- ○
- ○

TOOLS I USED:

- ○ Gua Sha
- ○ Microcurrent Device
- ○ Jade Roller
- ○ Ice Roller
- ○

8oz	8oz	8oz	8oz
8oz	8oz	8oz	8oz

WATER INTAKE

EVENING ROUTINE

TONIGHT MY SKIN FEELS:

TONIGHT I FEEL:

   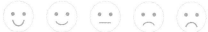

OTHER NOTES:

SKINCARE STEPS:

- ○ Cleanser
- ○ Toner
- ○ Spot Treatment
- ○ Serums
  - ○
  - ○
  - ○

- ○ Eye Cream
- ○ Moisturizer
- ○ Face Oil
- ○
- ○
- ○
- ○

where I'm breaking out

EXTRA STEPS:

- ○ Exfoliation
- ○ Retinol
- ○ Face Mask
- ○
- ○

- ○
- ○
- ○
- ○
- ○

OTHER NOTES:

routine tracker

MORNING ROUTINE

TODAY MY SKIN FEELS:

TODAY I FEEL:

  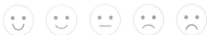

OTHER NOTES:

SKINCARE STEPS:

- ○ Cleanser
- ○ Toner
- ○ Spot Treatment
- ○ Serums
  - ○
  - ○
  - ○

- ○ Eye Cream
- ○ Moisturizer
- ○ Face Oil
- ○ Sunscreen
  - ○
  - ○
  - ○

where I'm breaking out

EXTRA STEPS:

- ○ Exfoliation
- ○ Face Mask
- ○ Face Massage
- ○
- ○

TOOLS I USED:

- ○ Gua Sha
- ○ Microcurrent Device
- ○ Jade Roller
- ○ Ice Roller
- ○

8oz	8oz	8oz	8oz
8oz	8oz	8oz	8oz

WATER INTAKE

weather:

sleep:

EVENING ROUTINE

TONIGHT MY SKIN FEELS:

TONIGHT I FEEL:

OTHER NOTES:

SKINCARE STEPS:

O Cleanser   O Eye Cream
O Toner   O Moisturizer
O Spot Treatment O Face Oil
O Serums   O
   O   O
   O   O
   O   O

where I'm breaking out

EXTRA STEPS: OTHER NOTES:

O Exfoliation   O
O Retinol   O
O Face Mask   O
O   O
O   O

routine tracker

MORNING ROUTINE

TODAY MY SKIN FEELS:

TODAY I FEEL:

  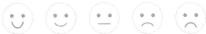

OTHER NOTES:

SKINCARE STEPS:

- ○ Cleanser
- ○ Toner
- ○ Spot Treatment
- ○ Serums
- ○
- ○
- ○

- ○ Eye Cream
- ○ Moisturizer
- ○ Face Oil
- ○ Sunscreen
- ○
- ○
- ○

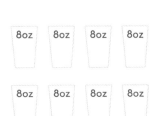

where I'm breaking out

EXTRA STEPS:

- ○ Exfoliation
- ○ Face Mask
- ○ Face Massage
- ○
- ○

TOOLS I USED:

- ○ Gua Sha
- ○ Microcurrent Device
- ○ Jade Roller
- ○ Ice Roller
- ○

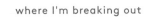

| 8oz | 8oz | 8oz | 8oz |
| 8oz | 8oz | 8oz | 8oz |

WATER INTAKE

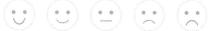
EVENING ROUTINE

TONIGHT MY SKIN FEELS:

TONIGHT I FEEL:

OTHER NOTES:

SKINCARE STEPS:

- ○ Cleanser
- ○ Toner
- ○ Spot Treatment
- ○ Serums
  - ○
  - ○
  - ○

- ○ Eye Cream
- ○ Moisturizer
- ○ Face Oil
- ○
- ○
- ○
- ○

where I'm breaking out

EXTRA STEPS:

- ○ Exfoliation
- ○ Retinol
- ○ Face Mask
- ○
- ○

- ○
- ○
- ○
- ○
- ○

OTHER NOTES:

routine tracker

MORNING ROUTINE

TODAY MY SKIN FEELS:

TODAY I FEEL:

   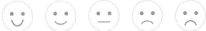

OTHER NOTES:

SKINCARE STEPS:

○ Cleanser   ○ Eye Cream
○ Toner   ○ Moisturizer
○ Spot Treatment ○ Face Oil
○ Serums   ○ Sunscreen
  ○   ○
  ○   ○
  ○   ○

where I'm breaking out

EXTRA STEPS: TOOLS I USED:

○ Exfoliation   ○ Gua Sha
○ Face Mask   ○ Microcurrent Device
○ Face Massage   ○ Jade Roller
○   ○ Ice Roller
○   ○

| 8oz | 8oz | 8oz | 8oz |
| 8oz | 8oz | 8oz | 8oz |

WATER INTAKE

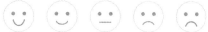
EVENING ROUTINE

TONIGHT MY SKIN FEELS:

TONIGHT I FEEL:

OTHER NOTES:

SKINCARE STEPS:

○ Cleanser   ○ Eye Cream
○ Toner   ○ Moisturizer
○ Spot Treatment ○ Face Oil
○ Serums   ○
　○   ○
　○   ○
　○   ○

where I'm breaking out

EXTRA STEPS: OTHER NOTES:

○ Exfoliation   ○
○ Retinol   ○
○ Face Mask   ○
○   ○
○   ○

routine tracker

MORNING ROUTINE

TODAY MY SKIN FEELS:

TODAY I FEEL:

OTHER NOTES:

SKINCARE STEPS:

○ Cleanser   ○ Eye Cream
○ Toner   ○ Moisturizer
○ Spot Treatment   ○ Face Oil
○ Serums   ○ Sunscreen
  ○   ○
  ○   ○
  ○ _____   ○ _____

where I'm breaking out

EXTRA STEPS: TOOLS I USED:

○ Exfoliation   ○ Gua Sha
○ Face Mask   ○ Microcurrent Device
○ Face Massage   ○ Jade Roller
○   ○ Ice Roller
○   ○

8oz	8oz	8oz	8oz
8oz	8oz	8oz	8oz

WATER INTAKE

EVENING ROUTINE

TONIGHT MY SKIN FEELS:

TONIGHT I FEEL:

OTHER NOTES:

SKINCARE STEPS:

○ Cleanser   ○ Eye Cream
○ Toner   ○ Moisturizer
○ Spot Treatment   ○ Face Oil
○ Serums   ○
   ○   ○
   ○   ○
   ○   ○

where I'm breaking out

EXTRA STEPS: OTHER NOTES:

○ Exfoliation   ○
○ Retinol   ○
○ Face Mask   ○
○   ○
○   ○

routine tracker

 date:

MORNING ROUTINE

TODAY MY SKIN FEELS:

TODAY I FEEL:

OTHER NOTES:

SKINCARE STEPS:

- ○ Cleanser
- ○ Toner
- ○ Spot Treatment
- ○ Serums
  - ○
  - ○
  - ○

- ○ Eye Cream
- ○ Moisturizer
- ○ Face Oil
- ○ Sunscreen
  - ○
  - ○
  - ○

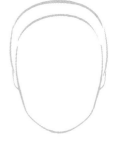

where I'm breaking out

EXTRA STEPS:

- ○ Exfoliation
- ○ Face Mask
- ○ Face Massage
- ○
- ○

TOOLS I USED:

- ○ Gua Sha
- ○ Microcurrent Device
- ○ Jade Roller
- ○ Ice Roller
- ○

| 8oz | 8oz | 8oz | 8oz |
| 8oz | 8oz | 8oz | 8oz |

WATER INTAKE

EVENING ROUTINE

TONIGHT MY SKIN FEELS:

TONIGHT I FEEL:

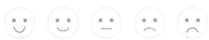

OTHER NOTES:

SKINCARE STEPS:

- ○ Cleanser
- ○ Toner
- ○ Spot Treatment
- ○ Serums
  - ○
  - ○
  - ○

- ○ Eye Cream
- ○ Moisturizer
- ○ Face Oil
- ○
- ○
- ○
- ○

where I'm breaking out

EXTRA STEPS:

OTHER NOTES:

- ○ Exfoliation
- ○ Retinol
- ○ Face Mask
- ○
- ○

- ○
- ○
- ○
- ○
- ○

routine tracker

MORNING ROUTINE

TODAY MY SKIN FEELS:

TODAY I FEEL:

OTHER NOTES:

SKINCARE STEPS:

- ○ Cleanser
- ○ Toner
- ○ Spot Treatment
- ○ Serums
- ○
- ○
- ○

- ○ Eye Cream
- ○ Moisturizer
- ○ Face Oil
- ○ Sunscreen
- ○
- ○
- ○

where I'm breaking out

EXTRA STEPS:

- ○ Exfoliation
- ○ Face Mask
- ○ Face Massage
- ○
- ○

TOOLS I USED:

- ○ Gua Sha
- ○ Microcurrent Device
- ○ Jade Roller
- ○ Ice Roller
- ○

8oz	8oz	8oz	8oz
8oz	8oz	8oz	8oz

WATER INTAKE

EVENING ROUTINE

TONIGHT MY SKIN FEELS:

TONIGHT I FEEL:

OTHER NOTES:

SKINCARE STEPS:

- ○ Cleanser
- ○ Toner
- ○ Spot Treatment
- ○ Serums
  - ○
  - ○
  - ○

- ○ Eye Cream
- ○ Moisturizer
- ○ Face Oil
- ○
- ○
- ○
- ○

where I'm breaking out

EXTRA STEPS:

- ○ Exfoliation
- ○ Retinol
- ○ Face Mask
- ○
- ○

- ○
- ○
- ○
- ○
- ○

OTHER NOTES:

routine tracker

MORNING ROUTINE

TODAY MY SKIN FEELS:

TODAY I FEEL:

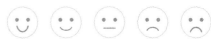

OTHER NOTES:

SKINCARE STEPS:

- ○ Cleanser
- ○ Toner
- ○ Spot Treatment
- ○ Serums
    - ○
    - ○
    - ○

- ○ Eye Cream
- ○ Moisturizer
- ○ Face Oil
- ○ Sunscreen
    - ○
    - ○
    - ○

where I'm breaking out

EXTRA STEPS:

- ○ Exfoliation
- ○ Face Mask
- ○ Face Massage
- ○
- ○

TOOLS I USED:

- ○ Gua Sha
- ○ Microcurrent Device
- ○ Jade Roller
- ○ Ice Roller
- ○

| 8oz | 8oz | 8oz | 8oz |
| 8oz | 8oz | 8oz | 8oz |

WATER INTAKE

EVENING ROUTINE

TONIGHT MY SKIN FEELS:

TONIGHT I FEEL:

OTHER NOTES:

SKINCARE STEPS:

- ○ Cleanser
- ○ Toner
- ○ Spot Treatment
- ○ Serums
  - ○
  - ○
  - ○

- ○ Eye Cream
- ○ Moisturizer
- ○ Face Oil
- ○
- ○
- ○
- ○

where I'm breaking out

EXTRA STEPS:

- ○ Exfoliation
- ○ Retinol
- ○ Face Mask
- ○
- ○

- ○
- ○
- ○
- ○
- ○

OTHER NOTES:

routine tracker

MORNING ROUTINE

TODAY MY SKIN FEELS:

TODAY I FEEL:

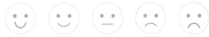

OTHER NOTES:

SKINCARE STEPS:

- ○ Cleanser
- ○ Toner
- ○ Spot Treatment
- ○ Serums
  - ○
  - ○
  - ○

- ○ Eye Cream
- ○ Moisturizer
- ○ Face Oil
- ○ Sunscreen
  - ○
  - ○
  - ○

where I'm breaking out

EXTRA STEPS:

- ○ Exfoliation
- ○ Face Mask
- ○ Face Massage
- ○
- ○

TOOLS I USED:

- ○ Gua Sha
- ○ Microcurrent Device
- ○ Jade Roller
- ○ Ice Roller
- ○

8oz	8oz	8oz	8oz
8oz	8oz	8oz	8oz

WATER INTAKE

EVENING ROUTINE

TONIGHT MY SKIN FEELS:

TONIGHT I FEEL:

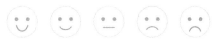

OTHER NOTES:

SKINCARE STEPS:

- ○ Cleanser
- ○ Toner
- ○ Spot Treatment
- ○ Serums
  - ○
  - ○
  - ○

- ○ Eye Cream
- ○ Moisturizer
- ○ Face Oil
- ○
- ○
- ○
- ○

where I'm breaking out

EXTRA STEPS:

- ○ Exfoliation
- ○ Retinol
- ○ Face Mask
- ○
- ○

- ○
- ○
- ○
- ○
- ○

OTHER NOTES:

routine tracker

 date:

MORNING ROUTINE

TODAY MY SKIN FEELS:

TODAY I FEEL:

  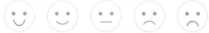

OTHER NOTES:

SKINCARE STEPS:

- ○ Cleanser
- ○ Toner
- ○ Spot Treatment
- ○ Serums
  - ○
  - ○
  - ○

- ○ Eye Cream
- ○ Moisturizer
- ○ Face Oil
- ○ Sunscreen
  - ○
  - ○
  - ○

where I'm breaking out

EXTRA STEPS:

- ○ Exfoliation
- ○ Face Mask
- ○ Face Massage
- ○
- ○

TOOLS I USED:

- ○ Gua Sha
- ○ Microcurrent Device
- ○ Jade Roller
- ○ Ice Roller
- ○

8oz	8oz	8oz	8oz
8oz	8oz	8oz	8oz

WATER INTAKE

EVENING ROUTINE

TONIGHT MY SKIN FEELS:

TONIGHT I FEEL:

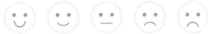

OTHER NOTES:

SKINCARE STEPS:

○ Cleanser   ○ Eye Cream
○ Toner   ○ Moisturizer
○ Spot Treatment   ○ Face Oil
○ Serums   ○
    ○   ○
    ○   ○
    ○   ○

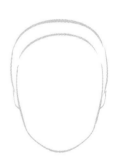

where I'm breaking out

EXTRA STEPS:

OTHER NOTES:

○ Exfoliation   ○
○ Retinol   ○
○ Face Mask   ○
○   ○
○   ○

routine tracker

MORNING ROUTINE

TODAY MY SKIN FEELS:

TODAY I FEEL:

OTHER NOTES:

SKINCARE STEPS:

- ○ Cleanser
- ○ Toner
- ○ Spot Treatment
- ○ Serums
  - ○
  - ○
  - ○
- ○ Eye Cream
- ○ Moisturizer
- ○ Face Oil
- ○ Sunscreen
  - ○
  - ○
  - ○

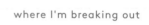

where I'm breaking out

EXTRA STEPS:

- ○ Exfoliation
- ○ Face Mask
- ○ Face Massage
- ○
- ○

TOOLS I USED:

- ○ Gua Sha
- ○ Microcurrent Device
- ○ Jade Roller
- ○ Ice Roller
- ○

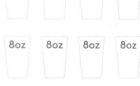

WATER INTAKE

EVENING ROUTINE

TONIGHT MY SKIN FEELS:

TONIGHT I FEEL:

OTHER NOTES:

SKINCARE STEPS:

○ Cleanser   ○ Eye Cream
○ Toner   ○ Moisturizer
○ Spot Treatment   ○ Face Oil
○ Serums   ○
    ○   ○
    ○   ○
    ○   ○

where I'm breaking out

EXTRA STEPS:

OTHER NOTES:

○ Exfoliation   ○
○ Retinol   ○
○ Face Mask   ○
○   ○
○   ○

routine tracker

MORNING ROUTINE

TODAY MY SKIN FEELS:

TODAY I FEEL:

   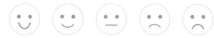

OTHER NOTES:

SKINCARE STEPS:

- ○ Cleanser
- ○ Toner
- ○ Spot Treatment
- ○ Serums
  - ○
  - ○
  - ○

- ○ Eye Cream
- ○ Moisturizer
- ○ Face Oil
- ○ Sunscreen
  - ○
  - ○
  - ○

where I'm breaking out

EXTRA STEPS:

- ○ Exfoliation
- ○ Face Mask
- ○ Face Massage
- ○
- ○

TOOLS I USED:

- ○ Gua Sha
- ○ Microcurrent Device
- ○ Jade Roller
- ○ Ice Roller
- ○

| 8oz | 8oz | 8oz | 8oz |
| 8oz | 8oz | 8oz | 8oz |

WATER INTAKE

EVENING ROUTINE

TONIGHT MY SKIN FEELS:

TONIGHT I FEEL:

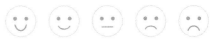

OTHER NOTES:

SKINCARE STEPS:

○ Cleanser   ○ Eye Cream

○ Toner   ○ Moisturizer

○ Spot Treatment   ○ Face Oil

○ Serums   ○

○   ○

○   ○

○   ○

where I'm breaking out

EXTRA STEPS:

OTHER NOTES:

○ Exfoliation   ○

○ Retinol   ○

○ Face Mask   ○

○   ○

○   ○

routine tracker

MORNING ROUTINE

TODAY MY SKIN FEELS:

TODAY I FEEL:

OTHER NOTES:

SKINCARE STEPS:

- ○ Cleanser
- ○ Toner
- ○ Spot Treatment
- ○ Serums
- ○
- ○
- ○

- ○ Eye Cream
- ○ Moisturizer
- ○ Face Oil
- ○ Sunscreen
- ○
- ○
- ○

where I'm breaking out

EXTRA STEPS:

- ○ Exfoliation
- ○ Face Mask
- ○ Face Massage
- ○
- ○

TOOLS I USED:

- ○ Gua Sha
- ○ Microcurrent Device
- ○ Jade Roller
- ○ Ice Roller
- ○

8oz	8oz	8oz	8oz
8oz	8oz	8oz	8oz

WATER INTAKE

EVENING ROUTINE

TONIGHT MY SKIN FEELS:

TONIGHT I FEEL:

OTHER NOTES:

SKINCARE STEPS:

○ Cleanser   ○ Eye Cream
○ Toner   ○ Moisturizer
○ Spot Treatment   ○ Face Oil
○ Serums   ○
    ○   ○
    ○   ○
    ○   ○

where I'm breaking out

EXTRA STEPS:

OTHER NOTES:

○ Exfoliation   ○
○ Retinol   ○
○ Face Mask   ○
○   ○
○   ○

routine tracker

 date:

TODAY MY SKIN FEELS:

TODAY I FEEL:

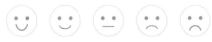

OTHER NOTES:

SKINCARE STEPS:

○ Cleanser   ○ Eye Cream
○ Toner   ○ Moisturizer
○ Spot Treatment   ○ Face Oil
○ Serums   ○ Sunscreen
   ○   ○
   ○   ○
   ○   ○

where I'm breaking out

EXTRA STEPS: TOOLS I USED:

○ Exfoliation   ○ Gua Sha
○ Face Mask   ○ Microcurrent Device
○ Face Massage   ○ Jade Roller
○   ○ Ice Roller
○   ○

8oz	8oz	8oz	8oz
8oz	8oz	8oz	8oz

WATER INTAKE

EVENING ROUTINE

TONIGHT MY SKIN FEELS:

TONIGHT I FEEL:

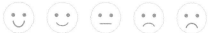

OTHER NOTES:

SKINCARE STEPS:

- ○ Cleanser
- ○ Toner
- ○ Spot Treatment
- ○ Serums
    - ○
    - ○
    - ○

- ○ Eye Cream
- ○ Moisturizer
- ○ Face Oil
- ○
- ○
- ○
- ○

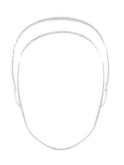

where I'm breaking out

EXTRA STEPS:

- ○ Exfoliation
- ○ Retinol
- ○ Face Mask
- ○
- ○

- ○
- ○
- ○
- ○
- ○

OTHER NOTES:

routine tracker

MORNING ROUTINE

TODAY MY SKIN FEELS:

TODAY I FEEL:

OTHER NOTES:

SKINCARE STEPS:

- ○ Cleanser
- ○ Toner
- ○ Spot Treatment
- ○ Serums
  - ○
  - ○
  - ○

- ○ Eye Cream
- ○ Moisturizer
- ○ Face Oil
- ○ Sunscreen
  - ○
  - ○
  - ○

where I'm breaking out

EXTRA STEPS:

- ○ Exfoliation
- ○ Face Mask
- ○ Face Massage
- ○
- ○

TOOLS I USED:

- ○ Gua Sha
- ○ Microcurrent Device
- ○ Jade Roller
- ○ Ice Roller
- ○

8oz	8oz	8oz	8oz
8oz	8oz	8oz	8oz

WATER INTAKE

EVENING ROUTINE

TONIGHT MY SKIN FEELS:

TONIGHT I FEEL:

OTHER NOTES:

SKINCARE STEPS:

- ○ Cleanser
- ○ Toner
- ○ Spot Treatment
- ○ Serums
    - ○
    - ○
    - ○

- ○ Eye Cream
- ○ Moisturizer
- ○ Face Oil
- ○
- ○
- ○
- ○

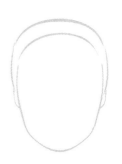

where I'm breaking out

EXTRA STEPS:

- ○ Exfoliation
- ○ Retinol
- ○ Face Mask
- ○
- ○

- ○
- ○
- ○
- ○
- ○

OTHER NOTES:

routine tracker

 date:

MORNING ROUTINE

TODAY MY SKIN FEELS:

TODAY I FEEL:

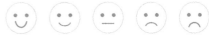

OTHER NOTES:

SKINCARE STEPS:

- ○ Cleanser
- ○ Toner
- ○ Spot Treatment
- ○ Serums
  - ○
  - ○
  - ○

- ○ Eye Cream
- ○ Moisturizer
- ○ Face Oil
- ○ Sunscreen
  - ○
  - ○
  - ○

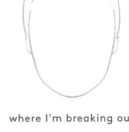

where I'm breaking out

EXTRA STEPS:

- ○ Exfoliation
- ○ Face Mask
- ○ Face Massage
- ○
- ○

TOOLS I USED:

- ○ Gua Sha
- ○ Microcurrent Device
- ○ Jade Roller
- ○ Ice Roller
- ○

| 8oz | 8oz | 8oz | 8oz |
| 8oz | 8oz | 8oz | 8oz |

WATER INTAKE

EVENING ROUTINE

TONIGHT MY SKIN FEELS:

TONIGHT I FEEL:

OTHER NOTES:

SKINCARE STEPS:

○ Cleanser   ○ Eye Cream
○ Toner   ○ Moisturizer
○ Spot Treatment   ○ Face Oil
○ Serums   ○
  ○   ○
  ○   ○
  ○   ○

where I'm breaking out

EXTRA STEPS:

OTHER NOTES:

○ Exfoliation   ○
○ Retinol   ○
○ Face Mask   ○
○   ○
○   ○

routine tracker

MORNING ROUTINE

TODAY MY SKIN FEELS:

TODAY I FEEL:

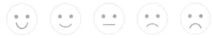

OTHER NOTES:

SKINCARE STEPS:

- ○ Cleanser
- ○ Toner
- ○ Spot Treatment
- ○ Serums
  - ○
  - ○
  - ○
- ○ Eye Cream
- ○ Moisturizer
- ○ Face Oil
- ○ Sunscreen
  - ○
  - ○
  - ○

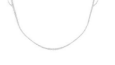

where I'm breaking out

EXTRA STEPS:

- ○ Exfoliation
- ○ Face Mask
- ○ Face Massage
- ○
- ○

TOOLS I USED:

- ○ Gua Sha
- ○ Microcurrent Device
- ○ Jade Roller
- ○ Ice Roller
- ○

8oz	8oz	8oz	8oz
8oz	8oz	8oz	8oz

WATER INTAKE

EVENING ROUTINE

TONIGHT MY SKIN FEELS:

TONIGHT I FEEL:

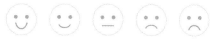

OTHER NOTES:

SKINCARE STEPS:

- ◯ Cleanser
- ◯ Toner
- ◯ Spot Treatment
- ◯ Serums
  - ◯
  - ◯
  - ◯

- ◯ Eye Cream
- ◯ Moisturizer
- ◯ Face Oil
- ◯
- ◯
- ◯
- ◯

where I'm breaking out

EXTRA STEPS:

- ◯ Exfoliation
- ◯ Retinol
- ◯ Face Mask
- ◯
- ◯

- ◯
- ◯
- ◯
- ◯
- ◯

OTHER NOTES:

routine tracker

MORNING ROUTINE

TODAY MY SKIN FEELS:

TODAY I FEEL:

 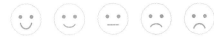

OTHER NOTES:

SKINCARE STEPS:

- ○ Cleanser
- ○ Toner
- ○ Spot Treatment
- ○ Serums
  - ○
  - ○
  - ○

- ○ Eye Cream
- ○ Moisturizer
- ○ Face Oil
- ○ Sunscreen
  - ○
  - ○
  - ○

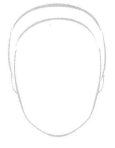

where I'm breaking out

EXTRA STEPS:

- ○ Exfoliation
- ○ Face Mask
- ○ Face Massage
- ○
- ○

TOOLS I USED:

- ○ Gua Sha
- ○ Microcurrent Device
- ○ Jade Roller
- ○ Ice Roller
- ○

| 8oz | 8oz | 8oz | 8oz |

| 8oz | 8oz | 8oz | 8oz |

WATER INTAKE

EVENING ROUTINE

TONIGHT MY SKIN FEELS:

TONIGHT I FEEL:

OTHER NOTES:

SKINCARE STEPS:

- ○ Cleanser
- ○ Toner
- ○ Spot Treatment
- ○ Serums
  - ○
  - ○
  - ○

- ○ Eye Cream
- ○ Moisturizer
- ○ Face Oil
- ○
- ○
- ○
- ○

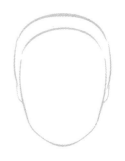

where I'm breaking out

EXTRA STEPS:

- ○ Exfoliation
- ○ Retinol
- ○ Face Mask
- ○
- ○

- ○
- ○
- ○
- ○
- ○

OTHER NOTES:

routine tracker

MORNING ROUTINE

TODAY MY SKIN FEELS:

TODAY I FEEL:

OTHER NOTES:

SKINCARE STEPS:

- ○ Cleanser
- ○ Toner
- ○ Spot Treatment
- ○ Serums
  - ○
  - ○
  - ○

- ○ Eye Cream
- ○ Moisturizer
- ○ Face Oil
- ○ Sunscreen
  - ○
  - ○
  - ○

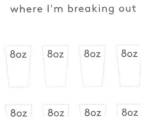

where I'm breaking out

EXTRA STEPS:

- ○ Exfoliation
- ○ Face Mask
- ○ Face Massage
- ○
- ○

TOOLS I USED:

- ○ Gua Sha
- ○ Microcurrent Device
- ○ Jade Roller
- ○ Ice Roller
- ○

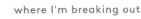

| 8oz | 8oz | 8oz | 8oz |
| 8oz | 8oz | 8oz | 8oz |

WATER INTAKE

EVENING ROUTINE

TONIGHT MY SKIN FEELS:

TONIGHT I FEEL:

OTHER NOTES:

SKINCARE STEPS:

- ○ Cleanser
- ○ Toner
- ○ Spot Treatment
- ○ Serums
    - ○
    - ○
    - ○

- ○ Eye Cream
- ○ Moisturizer
- ○ Face Oil
- ○
- ○
- ○
- ○

where I'm breaking out

EXTRA STEPS:

- ○ Exfoliation
- ○ Retinol
- ○ Face Mask
- ○
- ○

- ○
- ○
- ○
- ○
- ○

OTHER NOTES:

routine tracker

 date:

MORNING ROUTINE

TODAY MY SKIN FEELS:

TODAY I FEEL:

  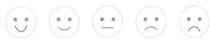

OTHER NOTES:

SKINCARE STEPS:

○ Cleanser
○ Toner
○ Spot Treatment
○ Serums
  ○
  ○
  ○

○ Eye Cream
○ Moisturizer
○ Face Oil
○ Sunscreen
  ○
  ○
  ○

where I'm breaking out

EXTRA STEPS:

○ Exfoliation
○ Face Mask
○ Face Massage
○
○

TOOLS I USED:

○ Gua Sha
○ Microcurrent Device
○ Jade Roller
○ Ice Roller
○

8oz	8oz	8oz	8oz
8oz	8oz	8oz	8oz

WATER INTAKE

EVENING ROUTINE

TONIGHT MY SKIN FEELS:

TONIGHT I FEEL:

OTHER NOTES:

SKINCARE STEPS:

- ○ Cleanser
- ○ Toner
- ○ Spot Treatment
- ○ Serums
- ○
- ○
- ○

- ○ Eye Cream
- ○ Moisturizer
- ○ Face Oil
- ○
- ○
- ○
- ○

where I'm breaking out

EXTRA STEPS:

- ○ Exfoliation
- ○ Retinol
- ○ Face Mask
- ○
- ○

- ○
- ○
- ○
- ○
- ○

OTHER NOTES:

routine tracker

MORNING ROUTINE

TODAY MY SKIN FEELS:

TODAY I FEEL:

OTHER NOTES:

SKINCARE STEPS:

- ○ Cleanser
- ○ Toner
- ○ Spot Treatment
- ○ Serums
  - ○
  - ○
  - ○

- ○ Eye Cream
- ○ Moisturizer
- ○ Face Oil
- ○ Sunscreen
  - ○
  - ○
  - ○

where I'm breaking out

EXTRA STEPS:

- ○ Exfoliation
- ○ Face Mask
- ○ Face Massage
- ○
- ○

TOOLS I USED:

- ○ Gua Sha
- ○ Microcurrent Device
- ○ Jade Roller
- ○ Ice Roller
- ○

| 8oz | 8oz | 8oz | 8oz |

| 8oz | 8oz | 8oz | 8oz |

WATER INTAKE

EVENING ROUTINE

TONIGHT MY SKIN FEELS:

TONIGHT I FEEL:

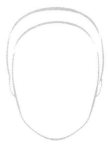

OTHER NOTES:

SKINCARE STEPS:

○ Cleanser   ○ Eye Cream
○ Toner   ○ Moisturizer
○ Spot Treatment   ○ Face Oil
○ Serums   ○
    ○   ○
    ○   ○
    ○   ○

where I'm breaking out

EXTRA STEPS: OTHER NOTES:

○ Exfoliation   ○
○ Retinol   ○
○ Face Mask   ○
○   ○
○   ○

routine tracker

 date:

MORNING ROUTINE

TODAY MY SKIN FEELS:

TODAY I FEEL:

OTHER NOTES:

SKINCARE STEPS:

- ⭘ Cleanser
- ⭘ Toner
- ⭘ Spot Treatment
- ⭘ Serums
- ⭘
- ⭘
- ⭘

- ⭘ Eye Cream
- ⭘ Moisturizer
- ⭘ Face Oil
- ⭘ Sunscreen
- ⭘
- ⭘
- ⭘

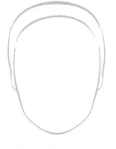

where I'm breaking out

EXTRA STEPS:

- ⭘ Exfoliation
- ⭘ Face Mask
- ⭘ Face Massage
- ⭘
- ⭘

TOOLS I USED:

- ⭘ Gua Sha
- ⭘ Microcurrent Device
- ⭘ Jade Roller
- ⭘ Ice Roller
- ⭘

8oz	8oz	8oz	8oz

8oz	8oz	8oz	8oz

WATER INTAKE

EVENING ROUTINE

TONIGHT MY SKIN FEELS:

TONIGHT I FEEL:

OTHER NOTES:

SKINCARE STEPS:

○ Cleanser   ○ Eye Cream
○ Toner   ○ Moisturizer
○ Spot Treatment   ○ Face Oil
○ Serums   ○
   ○   ○
   ○   ○
   ○   ○

where I'm breaking out

EXTRA STEPS:

○ Exfoliation   ○
○ Retinol   ○
○ Face Mask   ○
○   ○
○   ○

OTHER NOTES:

routine tracker

MORNING ROUTINE

TODAY MY SKIN FEELS:

TODAY I FEEL:

OTHER NOTES:

SKINCARE STEPS:

○ Cleanser
○ Toner
○ Spot Treatment
○ Serums
○
○
○

○ Eye Cream
○ Moisturizer
○ Face Oil
○ Sunscreen
○
○
○

where I'm breaking out

EXTRA STEPS:

○ Exfoliation
○ Face Mask
○ Face Massage
○
○

TOOLS I USED:

○ Gua Sha
○ Microcurrent Device
○ Jade Roller
○ Ice Roller
○

8oz	8oz	8oz	8oz
8oz	8oz	8oz	8oz

WATER INTAKE

EVENING ROUTINE

TONIGHT MY SKIN FEELS:

TONIGHT I FEEL:

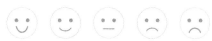

OTHER NOTES:

SKINCARE STEPS:

- ○ Cleanser
- ○ Toner
- ○ Spot Treatment
- ○ Serums
  - ○
  - ○
  - ○

- ○ Eye Cream
- ○ Moisturizer
- ○ Face Oil
- ○
- ○
- ○
- ○

where I'm breaking out

EXTRA STEPS:

- ○ Exfoliation
- ○ Retinol
- ○ Face Mask
- ○
- ○

- ○
- ○
- ○
- ○
- ○

OTHER NOTES:

routine tracker

MORNING ROUTINE

TODAY MY SKIN FEELS:

TODAY I FEEL:

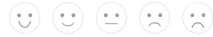

OTHER NOTES:

SKINCARE STEPS:

- ○ Cleanser
- ○ Toner
- ○ Spot Treatment
- ○ Serums
  - ○
  - ○
  - ○

- ○ Eye Cream
- ○ Moisturizer
- ○ Face Oil
- ○ Sunscreen
  - ○
  - ○
  - ○

where I'm breaking out

EXTRA STEPS:

- ○ Exfoliation
- ○ Face Mask
- ○ Face Massage
- ○
- ○

TOOLS I USED:

- ○ Gua Sha
- ○ Microcurrent Device
- ○ Jade Roller
- ○ Ice Roller
- ○

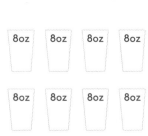

| 8oz | 8oz | 8oz | 8oz |
| 8oz | 8oz | 8oz | 8oz |

WATER INTAKE

EVENING ROUTINE

TONIGHT MY SKIN FEELS:

TONIGHT I FEEL:

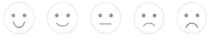

OTHER NOTES:

SKINCARE STEPS:

- ○ Cleanser
- ○ Toner
- ○ Spot Treatment
- ○ Serums
  - ○
  - ○
  - ○

- ○ Eye Cream
- ○ Moisturizer
- ○ Face Oil
- ○
- ○
- ○
- ○

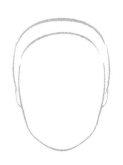

where I'm breaking out

EXTRA STEPS:

- ○ Exfoliation
- ○ Retinol
- ○ Face Mask
- ○
- ○

- ○
- ○
- ○
- ○
- ○

OTHER NOTES:

routine tracker

MORNING ROUTINE

TODAY MY SKIN FEELS:

TODAY I FEEL:

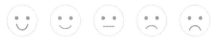

OTHER NOTES:

SKINCARE STEPS:

- ○ Cleanser
- ○ Toner
- ○ Spot Treatment
- ○ Serums
  - ○
  - ○
  - ○

- ○ Eye Cream
- ○ Moisturizer
- ○ Face Oil
- ○ Sunscreen
  - ○
  - ○
  - ○

where I'm breaking out

EXTRA STEPS:

- ○ Exfoliation
- ○ Face Mask
- ○ Face Massage
- ○
- ○

TOOLS I USED:

- ○ Gua Sha
- ○ Microcurrent Device
- ○ Jade Roller
- ○ Ice Roller
- ○

8oz	8oz	8oz	8oz
8oz	8oz	8oz	8oz

WATER INTAKE

EVENING ROUTINE

TONIGHT MY SKIN FEELS:

TONIGHT I FEEL:

OTHER NOTES:

SKINCARE STEPS:

- ○ Cleanser
- ○ Toner
- ○ Spot Treatment
- ○ Serums
  - ○
  - ○
  - ○

- ○ Eye Cream
- ○ Moisturizer
- ○ Face Oil
- ○
- ○
- ○
- ○

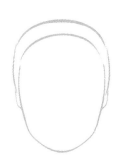

where I'm breaking out

EXTRA STEPS:

- ○ Exfoliation
- ○ Retinol
- ○ Face Mask
- ○
- ○

- ○
- ○
- ○
- ○
- ○

OTHER NOTES:

routine tracker

MORNING ROUTINE

TODAY MY SKIN FEELS:

TODAY I FEEL:

OTHER NOTES:

SKINCARE STEPS:

- ○ Cleanser
- ○ Toner
- ○ Spot Treatment
- ○ Serums
    - ○
    - ○
    - ○

- ○ Eye Cream
- ○ Moisturizer
- ○ Face Oil
- ○ Sunscreen
    - ○
    - ○
    - ○

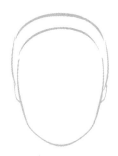

where I'm breaking out

EXTRA STEPS:

- ○ Exfoliation
- ○ Face Mask
- ○ Face Massage
- ○
- ○

TOOLS I USED:

- ○ Gua Sha
- ○ Microcurrent Device
- ○ Jade Roller
- ○ Ice Roller
- ○

8oz	8oz	8oz	8oz
8oz	8oz	8oz	8oz

WATER INTAKE

138

EVENING ROUTINE

TONIGHT MY SKIN FEELS:

TONIGHT I FEEL:

  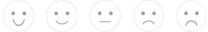

OTHER NOTES:

SKINCARE STEPS:

- ○ Cleanser
- ○ Toner
- ○ Spot Treatment
- ○ Serums
  - ○
  - ○
  - ○

- ○ Eye Cream
- ○ Moisturizer
- ○ Face Oil
- ○
- ○
- ○
- ○

where I'm breaking out

EXTRA STEPS:

- ○ Exfoliation
- ○ Retinol
- ○ Face Mask
- ○
- ○

- ○
- ○
- ○
- ○
- ○

OTHER NOTES:

routine tracker

MORNING ROUTINE

TODAY MY SKIN FEELS:

TODAY I FEEL:

OTHER NOTES:

SKINCARE STEPS:

- ○ Cleanser
- ○ Toner
- ○ Spot Treatment
- ○ Serums
  - ○
  - ○
  - ○
- ○ Eye Cream
- ○ Moisturizer
- ○ Face Oil
- ○ Sunscreen
  - ○
  - ○
  - ○

where I'm breaking out

EXTRA STEPS:

- ○ Exfoliation
- ○ Face Mask
- ○ Face Massage
- ○
- ○

TOOLS I USED:

- ○ Gua Sha
- ○ Microcurrent Device
- ○ Jade Roller
- ○ Ice Roller
- ○

8oz	8oz	8oz	8oz
8oz	8oz	8oz	8oz

WATER INTAKE

EVENING ROUTINE

TONIGHT MY SKIN FEELS:

TONIGHT I FEEL:

OTHER NOTES:

SKINCARE STEPS:

○ Cleanser   ○ Eye Cream
○ Toner   ○ Moisturizer
○ Spot Treatment   ○ Face Oil
○ Serums   ○
    ○   ○
    ○   ○
    ○   ○

where I'm breaking out

EXTRA STEPS: OTHER NOTES:

○ Exfoliation   ○
○ Retinol   ○
○ Face Mask   ○
○   ○
○   ○

routine tracker

MORNING ROUTINE

TODAY MY SKIN FEELS:

TODAY I FEEL:

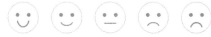

OTHER NOTES:

SKINCARE STEPS:

○ Cleanser   ○ Eye Cream
○ Toner   ○ Moisturizer
○ Spot Treatment   ○ Face Oil
○ Serums   ○ Sunscreen
  ○   ○
  ○   ○
  ○   ○

where I'm breaking out

EXTRA STEPS:

○ Exfoliation
○ Face Mask
○ Face Massage
○
○

TOOLS I USED:

○ Gua Sha
○ Microcurrent Device
○ Jade Roller
○ Ice Roller
○

8oz	8oz	8oz	8oz
8oz	8oz	8oz	8oz

WATER INTAKE

142

EVENING ROUTINE

TONIGHT MY SKIN FEELS:

TONIGHT I FEEL:

  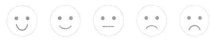

OTHER NOTES:

SKINCARE STEPS:

○ Cleanser   ○ Eye Cream
○ Toner   ○ Moisturizer
○ Spot Treatment ○ Face Oil
○ Serums   ○
   ○   ○
   ○   ○
   ○   ○

where I'm breaking out

EXTRA STEPS: OTHER NOTES:

○ Exfoliation   ○
○ Retinol   ○
○ Face Mask   ○
○   ○
○   ○

routine tracker

MORNING ROUTINE

TODAY MY SKIN FEELS:

TODAY I FEEL:

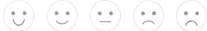

OTHER NOTES:

SKINCARE STEPS:

- ○ Cleanser
- ○ Toner
- ○ Spot Treatment
- ○ Serums
  - ○
  - ○
  - ○
- ○ Eye Cream
- ○ Moisturizer
- ○ Face Oil
- ○ Sunscreen
  - ○
  - ○
  - ○

where I'm breaking out

EXTRA STEPS:

- ○ Exfoliation
- ○ Face Mask
- ○ Face Massage
- ○
- ○

TOOLS I USED:

- ○ Gua Sha
- ○ Microcurrent Device
- ○ Jade Roller
- ○ Ice Roller
- ○

8oz	8oz	8oz	8oz
8oz	8oz	8oz	8oz

WATER INTAKE

EVENING ROUTINE

TONIGHT MY SKIN FEELS:

OTHER NOTES:

TONIGHT I FEEL:

SKINCARE STEPS:

- ○ Cleanser
- ○ Toner
- ○ Spot Treatment
- ○ Serums
  - ○
  - ○
  - ○

- ○ Eye Cream
- ○ Moisturizer
- ○ Face Oil
- ○
- ○
- ○
- ○

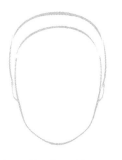

where I'm breaking out

EXTRA STEPS:

- ○ Exfoliation
- ○ Retinol
- ○ Face Mask
- ○
- ○

- ○
- ○
- ○
- ○
- ○

OTHER NOTES:

routine tracker

MORNING ROUTINE

TODAY MY SKIN FEELS:

TODAY I FEEL:

  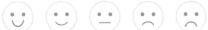

OTHER NOTES:

SKINCARE STEPS:

- ○ Cleanser
- ○ Toner
- ○ Spot Treatment
- ○ Serums
  - ○
  - ○
  - ○

- ○ Eye Cream
- ○ Moisturizer
- ○ Face Oil
- ○ Sunscreen
  - ○
  - ○
  - ○

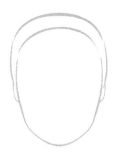

where I'm breaking out

EXTRA STEPS:

- ○ Exfoliation
- ○ Face Mask
- ○ Face Massage
- ○
- ○

TOOLS I USED:

- ○ Gua Sha
- ○ Microcurrent Device
- ○ Jade Roller
- ○ Ice Roller
- ○

8oz	8oz	8oz	8oz
8oz	8oz	8oz	8oz

WATER INTAKE

EVENING ROUTINE

TONIGHT MY SKIN FEELS:

TONIGHT I FEEL:

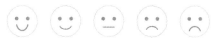

OTHER NOTES:

SKINCARE STEPS:

○ Cleanser   ○ Eye Cream
○ Toner   ○ Moisturizer
○ Spot Treatment   ○ Face Oil
○ Serums   ○
○   ○
○   ○
○   ○

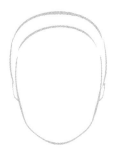

where I'm breaking out

EXTRA STEPS:

○ Exfoliation   ○
○ Retinol   ○
○ Face Mask   ○
○   ○
○   ○

OTHER NOTES:

routine tracker

MORNING ROUTINE

TODAY MY SKIN FEELS:

TODAY I FEEL:

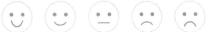

OTHER NOTES:

SKINCARE STEPS:

- ○ Cleanser
- ○ Toner
- ○ Spot Treatment
- ○ Serums
  - ○
  - ○
  - ○

- ○ Eye Cream
- ○ Moisturizer
- ○ Face Oil
- ○ Sunscreen
  - ○
  - ○
  - ○

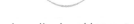

where I'm breaking out

EXTRA STEPS:

- ○ Exfoliation
- ○ Face Mask
- ○ Face Massage
- ○
- ○

TOOLS I USED:

- ○ Gua Sha
- ○ Microcurrent Device
- ○ Jade Roller
- ○ Ice Roller
- ○

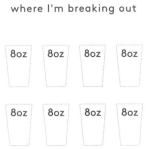

WATER INTAKE

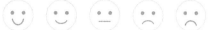
EVENING ROUTINE

TONIGHT MY SKIN FEELS:

TONIGHT I FEEL:

OTHER NOTES:

SKINCARE STEPS:

○ Cleanser   ○ Eye Cream
○ Toner   ○ Moisturizer
○ Spot Treatment   ○ Face Oil
○ Serums   ○
  ○   ○
  ○   ○
  ○   ○

where I'm breaking out

EXTRA STEPS: OTHER NOTES:

○ Exfoliation   ○
○ Retinol   ○
○ Face Mask   ○
○   ○
○   ○

routine tracker

MORNING ROUTINE

TODAY MY SKIN FEELS:

TODAY I FEEL:

  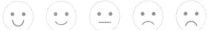

OTHER NOTES:

SKINCARE STEPS:

- ○ Cleanser
- ○ Toner
- ○ Spot Treatment
- ○ Serums
  - ○
  - ○
  - ○

- ○ Eye Cream
- ○ Moisturizer
- ○ Face Oil
- ○ Sunscreen
  - ○
  - ○
  - ○

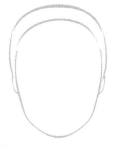

where I'm breaking out

EXTRA STEPS:

- ○ Exfoliation
- ○ Face Mask
- ○ Face Massage
- ○
- ○

TOOLS I USED:

- ○ Gua Sha
- ○ Microcurrent Device
- ○ Jade Roller
- ○ Ice Roller
- ○

8oz | 8oz | 8oz | 8oz

8oz | 8oz | 8oz | 8oz

WATER INTAKE

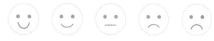

EVENING ROUTINE

TONIGHT MY SKIN FEELS:

TONIGHT I FEEL:

OTHER NOTES:

SKINCARE STEPS:

- ○ Cleanser
- ○ Toner
- ○ Spot Treatment
- ○ Serums
  - ○
  - ○
  - ○

- ○ Eye Cream
- ○ Moisturizer
- ○ Face Oil
- ○
- ○
- ○
- ○

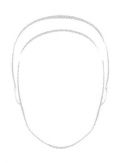

where I'm breaking out

EXTRA STEPS:

- ○ Exfoliation
- ○ Retinol
- ○ Face Mask
- ○
- ○

- ○
- ○
- ○
- ○
- ○

OTHER NOTES:

routine tracker

 date:

MORNING ROUTINE

TODAY MY SKIN FEELS:

TODAY I FEEL:

OTHER NOTES:

SKINCARE STEPS:

○ Cleanser   ○ Eye Cream
○ Toner   ○ Moisturizer
○ Spot Treatment   ○ Face Oil
○ Serums   ○ Sunscreen
   ○   ○
   ○   ○
   ○   ○

where I'm breaking out

EXTRA STEPS:

○ Exfoliation
○ Face Mask
○ Face Massage
○
○

TOOLS I USED:

○ Gua Sha
○ Microcurrent Device
○ Jade Roller
○ Ice Roller
○

| 8oz | 8oz | 8oz | 8oz |
| 8oz | 8oz | 8oz | 8oz |

WATER INTAKE

EVENING ROUTINE

TONIGHT MY SKIN FEELS:

TONIGHT I FEEL:

OTHER NOTES:

SKINCARE STEPS:

- ○ Cleanser
- ○ Toner
- ○ Spot Treatment
- ○ Serums
- ○
- ○
- ○

- ○ Eye Cream
- ○ Moisturizer
- ○ Face Oil
- ○
- ○
- ○
- ○

where I'm breaking out

EXTRA STEPS:

- ○ Exfoliation
- ○ Retinol
- ○ Face Mask
- ○
- ○

- ○
- ○
- ○
- ○
- ○

OTHER NOTES:

routine tracker

MORNING ROUTINE

TODAY MY SKIN FEELS:

TODAY I FEEL:

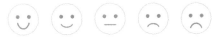

OTHER NOTES:

SKINCARE STEPS:

- ○ Cleanser
- ○ Toner
- ○ Spot Treatment
- ○ Serums
  - ○
  - ○
  - ○

- ○ Eye Cream
- ○ Moisturizer
- ○ Face Oil
- ○ Sunscreen
  - ○
  - ○
  - ○

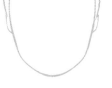

where I'm breaking out

EXTRA STEPS:

- ○ Exfoliation
- ○ Face Mask
- ○ Face Massage
- ○
- ○

TOOLS I USED:

- ○ Gua Sha
- ○ Microcurrent Device
- ○ Jade Roller
- ○ Ice Roller
- ○

WATER INTAKE

EVENING ROUTINE

TONIGHT MY SKIN FEELS:

TONIGHT I FEEL:

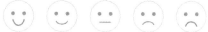

OTHER NOTES:

SKINCARE STEPS:

○ Cleanser ○ Eye Cream
○ Toner ○ Moisturizer
○ Spot Treatment ○ Face Oil
○ Serums ○
   ○ ○
   ○ ○
   ○ ○

where I'm breaking out

EXTRA STEPS:

○ Exfoliation ○
○ Retinol ○
○ Face Mask ○
○ ○
○ ○

OTHER NOTES:

routine tracker

MORNING ROUTINE

TODAY MY SKIN FEELS:

TODAY I FEEL:

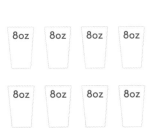

OTHER NOTES:

SKINCARE STEPS:

- ○ Cleanser
- ○ Toner
- ○ Spot Treatment
- ○ Serums
  - ○
  - ○
  - ○

- ○ Eye Cream
- ○ Moisturizer
- ○ Face Oil
- ○ Sunscreen
  - ○
  - ○
  - ○

where I'm breaking out

EXTRA STEPS:

- ○ Exfoliation
- ○ Face Mask
- ○ Face Massage
- ○
- ○

TOOLS I USED:

- ○ Gua Sha
- ○ Microcurrent Device
- ○ Jade Roller
- ○ Ice Roller
- ○

8oz	8oz	8oz	8oz
8oz	8oz	8oz	8oz

WATER INTAKE

EVENING ROUTINE

TONIGHT MY SKIN FEELS:

TONIGHT I FEEL:

OTHER NOTES:

SKINCARE STEPS:

- ○ Cleanser
- ○ Toner
- ○ Spot Treatment
- ○ Serums
- ○
- ○
- ○

- ○ Eye Cream
- ○ Moisturizer
- ○ Face Oil
- ○
- ○
- ○
- ○

where I'm breaking out

EXTRA STEPS:

- ○ Exfoliation
- ○ Retinol
- ○ Face Mask
- ○
- ○

- ○
- ○
- ○
- ○
- ○

OTHER NOTES:

routine tracker

date:

MORNING ROUTINE

TODAY MY SKIN FEELS:

TODAY I FEEL:

   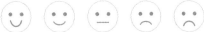

OTHER NOTES:

SKINCARE STEPS:

- ○ Cleanser
- ○ Toner
- ○ Spot Treatment
- ○ Serums
  - ○
  - ○
  - ○

- ○ Eye Cream
- ○ Moisturizer
- ○ Face Oil
- ○ Sunscreen
  - ○
  - ○
  - ○

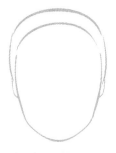

where I'm breaking out

EXTRA STEPS:

- ○ Exfoliation
- ○ Face Mask
- ○ Face Massage
- ○
- ○

TOOLS I USED:

- ○ Gua Sha
- ○ Microcurrent Device
- ○ Jade Roller
- ○ Ice Roller
- ○

8oz	8oz	8oz	8oz
8oz	8oz	8oz	8oz

WATER INTAKE

weather:

sleep:

EVENING ROUTINE

TONIGHT MY SKIN FEELS:

TONIGHT I FEEL:

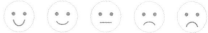

OTHER NOTES:

SKINCARE STEPS:

- ○ Cleanser
- ○ Toner
- ○ Spot Treatment
- ○ Serums
  - ○
  - ○
  - ○

- ○ Eye Cream
- ○ Moisturizer
- ○ Face Oil
- ○
- ○
- ○
- ○

where I'm breaking out

EXTRA STEPS:

- ○ Exfoliation
- ○ Retinol
- ○ Face Mask
- ○
- ○

- ○
- ○
- ○
- ○
- ○

OTHER NOTES:

routine tracker

MORNING ROUTINE

TODAY MY SKIN FEELS:

TODAY I FEEL:

OTHER NOTES:

SKINCARE STEPS:

- ○ Cleanser
- ○ Toner
- ○ Spot Treatment
- ○ Serums
  - ○
  - ○
  - ○

- ○ Eye Cream
- ○ Moisturizer
- ○ Face Oil
- ○ Sunscreen
  - ○
  - ○
  - ○

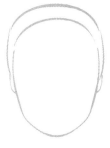

where I'm breaking out

EXTRA STEPS:

- ○ Exfoliation
- ○ Face Mask
- ○ Face Massage
- ○
- ○

TOOLS I USED:

- ○ Gua Sha
- ○ Microcurrent Device
- ○ Jade Roller
- ○ Ice Roller
- ○

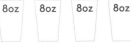

| 8oz | 8oz | 8oz | 8oz |
| 8oz | 8oz | 8oz | 8oz |

WATER INTAKE

EVENING ROUTINE

TONIGHT MY SKIN FEELS:

TONIGHT I FEEL:

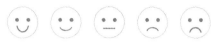

OTHER NOTES:

SKINCARE STEPS:

- ○ Cleanser
- ○ Toner
- ○ Spot Treatment
- ○ Serums
  - ○
  - ○
  - ○

- ○ Eye Cream
- ○ Moisturizer
- ○ Face Oil
- ○
- ○
- ○
- ○

where I'm breaking out

EXTRA STEPS:

- ○ Exfoliation
- ○ Retinol
- ○ Face Mask
- ○
- ○

- ○
- ○
- ○
- ○
- ○

OTHER NOTES:

routine tracker

MORNING ROUTINE

TODAY MY SKIN FEELS:

TODAY I FEEL:

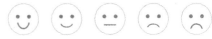

OTHER NOTES:

SKINCARE STEPS:

- ○ Cleanser
- ○ Toner
- ○ Spot Treatment
- ○ Serums
  - ○
  - ○
  - ○

- ○ Eye Cream
- ○ Moisturizer
- ○ Face Oil
- ○ Sunscreen
  - ○
  - ○
  - ○

where I'm breaking out

EXTRA STEPS:

- ○ Exfoliation
- ○ Face Mask
- ○ Face Massage
- ○
- ○

TOOLS I USED:

- ○ Gua Sha
- ○ Microcurrent Device
- ○ Jade Roller
- ○ Ice Roller
- ○

8oz	8oz	8oz	8oz
8oz	8oz	8oz	8oz

WATER INTAKE

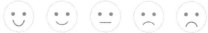
EVENING ROUTINE

TONIGHT MY SKIN FEELS:

TONIGHT I FEEL:

☺ ☺ 😐 ☹ ☹

OTHER NOTES:

SKINCARE STEPS:

- ○ Cleanser
- ○ Toner
- ○ Spot Treatment
- ○ Serums
  - ○
  - ○
  - ○

- ○ Eye Cream
- ○ Moisturizer
- ○ Face Oil
- ○
- ○
- ○
- ○

where I'm breaking out

EXTRA STEPS:

- ○ Exfoliation
- ○ Retinol
- ○ Face Mask
- ○
- ○

- ○
- ○
- ○
- ○
- ○

OTHER NOTES:

routine tracker

 date:

MORNING ROUTINE

TODAY MY SKIN FEELS:

TODAY I FEEL:

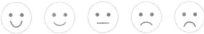

OTHER NOTES:

SKINCARE STEPS:

- ○ Cleanser
- ○ Toner
- ○ Spot Treatment
- ○ Serums
  - ○
  - ○
  - ○

- ○ Eye Cream
- ○ Moisturizer
- ○ Face Oil
- ○ Sunscreen
  - ○
  - ○
  - ○

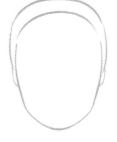

where I'm breaking out

EXTRA STEPS:

- ○ Exfoliation
- ○ Face Mask
- ○ Face Massage
- ○
- ○

TOOLS I USED:

- ○ Gua Sha
- ○ Microcurrent Device
- ○ Jade Roller
- ○ Ice Roller
- ○

8oz	8oz	8oz	8oz
8oz	8oz	8oz	8oz

WATER INTAKE

EVENING ROUTINE

TONIGHT MY SKIN FEELS:

TONIGHT I FEEL:

OTHER NOTES:

SKINCARE STEPS:

- ○ Cleanser
- ○ Toner
- ○ Spot Treatment
- ○ Serums
  - ○
  - ○
  - ○

- ○ Eye Cream
- ○ Moisturizer
- ○ Face Oil
- ○
- ○
- ○
- ○

where I'm breaking out

EXTRA STEPS:

- ○ Exfoliation
- ○ Retinol
- ○ Face Mask
- ○
- ○

- ○
- ○
- ○
- ○
- ○

OTHER NOTES:

routine tracker

 date:

MORNING ROUTINE

TODAY MY SKIN FEELS:

TODAY I FEEL:

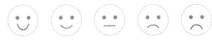

OTHER NOTES:

SKINCARE STEPS:

- ○ Cleanser
- ○ Toner
- ○ Spot Treatment
- ○ Serums
  - ○
  - ○
  - ○

- ○ Eye Cream
- ○ Moisturizer
- ○ Face Oil
- ○ Sunscreen
  - ○
  - ○
  - ○

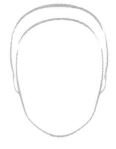

where I'm breaking out

EXTRA STEPS:

- ○ Exfoliation
- ○ Face Mask
- ○ Face Massage
- ○
- ○

TOOLS I USED:

- ○ Gua Sha
- ○ Microcurrent Device
- ○ Jade Roller
- ○ Ice Roller
- ○

| 8oz | 8oz | 8oz | 8oz |
| 8oz | 8oz | 8oz | 8oz |

WATER INTAKE

EVENING ROUTINE

TONIGHT MY SKIN FEELS:

TONIGHT I FEEL:

    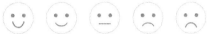

OTHER NOTES:

SKINCARE STEPS:

- ○ Cleanser
- ○ Toner
- ○ Spot Treatment
- ○ Serums
  - ○
  - ○
  - ○

- ○ Eye Cream
- ○ Moisturizer
- ○ Face Oil
- ○
- ○
- ○
- ○

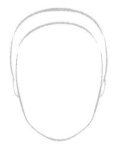

where I'm breaking out

EXTRA STEPS:

- ○ Exfoliation
- ○ Retinol
- ○ Face Mask
- ○
- ○

- ○
- ○
- ○
- ○
- ○

OTHER NOTES:

routine tracker

MORNING ROUTINE

TODAY MY SKIN FEELS:

TODAY I FEEL:

OTHER NOTES:

SKINCARE STEPS:

- ○ Cleanser
- ○ Toner
- ○ Spot Treatment
- ○ Serums
  - ○
  - ○
  - ○

- ○ Eye Cream
- ○ Moisturizer
- ○ Face Oil
- ○ Sunscreen
  - ○
  - ○
  - ○

where I'm breaking out

EXTRA STEPS:

- ○ Exfoliation
- ○ Face Mask
- ○ Face Massage
- ○
- ○

TOOLS I USED:

- ○ Gua Sha
- ○ Microcurrent Device
- ○ Jade Roller
- ○ Ice Roller
- ○

| 8oz | 8oz | 8oz | 8oz |
| 8oz | 8oz | 8oz | 8oz |

WATER INTAKE

EVENING ROUTINE

TONIGHT MY SKIN FEELS:

TONIGHT I FEEL:

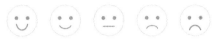

OTHER NOTES:

SKINCARE STEPS:

○ Cleanser   ○ Eye Cream
○ Toner   ○ Moisturizer
○ Spot Treatment ○ Face Oil
○ Serums   ○
    ○   ○
    ○   ○
    ○   ○

where I'm breaking out

EXTRA STEPS:

OTHER NOTES:

○ Exfoliation   ○
○ Retinol   ○
○ Face Mask   ○
○   ○
○   ○

routine tracker

MORNING ROUTINE

TODAY MY SKIN FEELS:

TODAY I FEEL:

   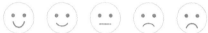

OTHER NOTES:

SKINCARE STEPS:

- ○ Cleanser
- ○ Toner
- ○ Spot Treatment
- ○ Serums
    - ○
    - ○
    - ○
- ○ Eye Cream
- ○ Moisturizer
- ○ Face Oil
- ○ Sunscreen
    - ○
    - ○
    - ○

where I'm breaking out

EXTRA STEPS:

- ○ Exfoliation
- ○ Face Mask
- ○ Face Massage
- ○
- ○

TOOLS I USED:

- ○ Gua Sha
- ○ Microcurrent Device
- ○ Jade Roller
- ○ Ice Roller
- ○

| 8oz | 8oz | 8oz | 8oz |
| 8oz | 8oz | 8oz | 8oz |

WATER INTAKE

EVENING ROUTINE

TONIGHT MY SKIN FEELS:

TONIGHT I FEEL:

OTHER NOTES:

SKINCARE STEPS:

- ○ Cleanser
- ○ Toner
- ○ Spot Treatment
- ○ Serums
  - ○
  - ○
  - ○

- ○ Eye Cream
- ○ Moisturizer
- ○ Face Oil
- ○
- ○
- ○
- ○

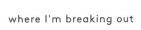

where I'm breaking out

EXTRA STEPS:

- ○ Exfoliation
- ○ Retinol
- ○ Face Mask
- ○
- ○

- ○
- ○
- ○
- ○
- ○

OTHER NOTES:

routine tracker

MORNING ROUTINE

TODAY MY SKIN FEELS:

TODAY I FEEL:

OTHER NOTES:

SKINCARE STEPS:

- ○ Cleanser
- ○ Toner
- ○ Spot Treatment
- ○ Serums
  - ○
  - ○
  - ○

- ○ Eye Cream
- ○ Moisturizer
- ○ Face Oil
- ○ Sunscreen
  - ○
  - ○
  - ○

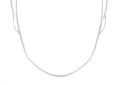

where I'm breaking out

EXTRA STEPS:

- ○ Exfoliation
- ○ Face Mask
- ○ Face Massage
- ○
- ○

TOOLS I USED:

- ○ Gua Sha
- ○ Microcurrent Device
- ○ Jade Roller
- ○ Ice Roller
- ○

8oz	8oz	8oz	8oz
8oz	8oz	8oz	8oz

WATER INTAKE

EVENING ROUTINE

TONIGHT MY SKIN FEELS:

TONIGHT I FEEL:

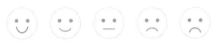

OTHER NOTES:

SKINCARE STEPS:

- ○ Cleanser
- ○ Toner
- ○ Spot Treatment
- ○ Serums
  - ○
  - ○
  - ○

- ○ Eye Cream
- ○ Moisturizer
- ○ Face Oil
- ○
- ○
- ○
- ○

where I'm breaking out

EXTRA STEPS:

- ○ Exfoliation
- ○ Retinol
- ○ Face Mask
- ○
- ○

- ○
- ○
- ○
- ○
- ○

OTHER NOTES:

routine tracker

MORNING ROUTINE

TODAY MY SKIN FEELS:

TODAY I FEEL:

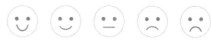

OTHER NOTES:

SKINCARE STEPS:

- ○ Cleanser
- ○ Toner
- ○ Spot Treatment
- ○ Serums
    - ○
    - ○
    - ○

- ○ Eye Cream
- ○ Moisturizer
- ○ Face Oil
- ○ Sunscreen
    - ○
    - ○
    - ○

where I'm breaking out

EXTRA STEPS:

- ○ Exfoliation
- ○ Face Mask
- ○ Face Massage
- ○
- ○

TOOLS I USED:

- ○ Gua Sha
- ○ Microcurrent Device
- ○ Jade Roller
- ○ Ice Roller
- ○

8oz	8oz	8oz	8oz
8oz	8oz	8oz	8oz

WATER INTAKE

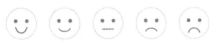

EVENING ROUTINE

TONIGHT MY SKIN FEELS:

TONIGHT I FEEL:

OTHER NOTES:

SKINCARE STEPS:

○ Cleanser   ○ Eye Cream
○ Toner   ○ Moisturizer
○ Spot Treatment ○ Face Oil
○ Serums   ○
   ○   ○
   ○   ○
   ○   ○

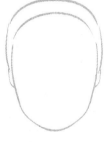

where I'm breaking out

EXTRA STEPS:

○ Exfoliation   ○
○ Retinol   ○
○ Face Mask   ○
○   ○
○   ○

OTHER NOTES:

routine tracker

MORNING ROUTINE

TODAY MY SKIN FEELS:

TODAY I FEEL:

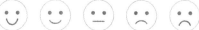

OTHER NOTES:

SKINCARE STEPS:

- ○ Cleanser
- ○ Toner
- ○ Spot Treatment
- ○ Serums
  - ○
  - ○
  - ○

- ○ Eye Cream
- ○ Moisturizer
- ○ Face Oil
- ○ Sunscreen
  - ○
  - ○
  - ○

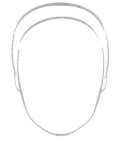

where I'm breaking out

EXTRA STEPS:

- ○ Exfoliation
- ○ Face Mask
- ○ Face Massage
- ○
- ○

TOOLS I USED:

- ○ Gua Sha
- ○ Microcurrent Device
- ○ Jade Roller
- ○ Ice Roller
- ○

| 8oz | 8oz | 8oz | 8oz |
| 8oz | 8oz | 8oz | 8oz |

WATER INTAKE

EVENING ROUTINE

TONIGHT MY SKIN FEELS:

TONIGHT I FEEL:

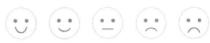

OTHER NOTES:

SKINCARE STEPS:

○ Cleanser   ○ Eye Cream
○ Toner   ○ Moisturizer
○ Spot Treatment ○ Face Oil
○ Serums   ○
   ○   ○
   ○   ○
   ○   ○

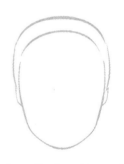

where I'm breaking out

EXTRA STEPS: OTHER NOTES:

○ Exfoliation   ○
○ Retinol   ○
○ Face Mask   ○
○   ○
○   ○

routine tracker

 date:

MORNING ROUTINE

TODAY MY SKIN FEELS:

TODAY I FEEL:

OTHER NOTES:

SKINCARE STEPS:

- ○ Cleanser
- ○ Toner
- ○ Spot Treatment
- ○ Serums
    - ○
    - ○
    - ○

- ○ Eye Cream
- ○ Moisturizer
- ○ Face Oil
- ○ Sunscreen
    - ○
    - ○
    - ○

where I'm breaking out

EXTRA STEPS:

- ○ Exfoliation
- ○ Face Mask
- ○ Face Massage
- ○
- ○

TOOLS I USED:

- ○ Gua Sha
- ○ Microcurrent Device
- ○ Jade Roller
- ○ Ice Roller
- ○

| 8oz | 8oz | 8oz | 8oz |
| 8oz | 8oz | 8oz | 8oz |

WATER INTAKE

EVENING ROUTINE

TONIGHT MY SKIN FEELS:

TONIGHT I FEEL:

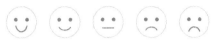

OTHER NOTES:

SKINCARE STEPS:

- O Cleanser
- O Toner
- O Spot Treatment
- O Serums
  - O
  - O
  - O

- O Eye Cream
- O Moisturizer
- O Face Oil
- O
- O
- O
- O
- O

where I'm breaking out

EXTRA STEPS:

- O Exfoliation
- O Retinol
- O Face Mask
- O
- O

- O
- O
- O
- O
- O

OTHER NOTES:

routine tracker

 date:

MORNING ROUTINE

TODAY MY SKIN FEELS:

TODAY I FEEL:

  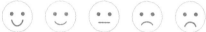

OTHER NOTES:

SKINCARE STEPS:

- ○ Cleanser
- ○ Toner
- ○ Spot Treatment
- ○ Serums
  - ○
  - ○
  - ○

- ○ Eye Cream
- ○ Moisturizer
- ○ Face Oil
- ○ Sunscreen
  - ○
  - ○
  - ○

where I'm breaking out

EXTRA STEPS:

- ○ Exfoliation
- ○ Face Mask
- ○ Face Massage
- ○
- ○

TOOLS I USED:

- ○ Gua Sha
- ○ Microcurrent Device
- ○ Jade Roller
- ○ Ice Roller
- ○

8oz	8oz	8oz	8oz
8oz	8oz	8oz	8oz

WATER INTAKE

EVENING ROUTINE

TONIGHT MY SKIN FEELS:

TONIGHT I FEEL:

OTHER NOTES:

SKINCARE STEPS:

- ○ Cleanser
- ○ Toner
- ○ Spot Treatment
- ○ Serums
  - ○
  - ○
  - ○

- ○ Eye Cream
- ○ Moisturizer
- ○ Face Oil
- ○
- ○
- ○
- ○

where I'm breaking out

EXTRA STEPS:

- ○ Exfoliation
- ○ Retinol
- ○ Face Mask
- ○
- ○

- ○
- ○
- ○
- ○
- ○

OTHER NOTES:

181

routine tracker

MORNING ROUTINE

TODAY MY SKIN FEELS:

TODAY I FEEL:

  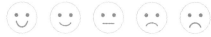

OTHER NOTES:

SKINCARE STEPS:

- ○ Cleanser
- ○ Toner
- ○ Spot Treatment
- ○ Serums
  - ○
  - ○
  - ○

- ○ Eye Cream
- ○ Moisturizer
- ○ Face Oil
- ○ Sunscreen
  - ○
  - ○
  - ○

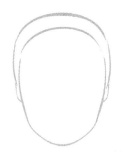

where I'm breaking out

EXTRA STEPS:

- ○ Exfoliation
- ○ Face Mask
- ○ Face Massage
- ○
- ○

TOOLS I USED:

- ○ Gua Sha
- ○ Microcurrent Device
- ○ Jade Roller
- ○ Ice Roller
- ○

8oz	8oz	8oz	8oz
8oz	8oz	8oz	8oz

WATER INTAKE

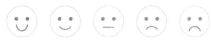

EVENING ROUTINE

TONIGHT MY SKIN FEELS:

TONIGHT I FEEL:

OTHER NOTES:

SKINCARE STEPS:

- ○ Cleanser
- ○ Toner
- ○ Spot Treatment
- ○ Serums
  - ○
  - ○
  - ○

- ○ Eye Cream
- ○ Moisturizer
- ○ Face Oil
- ○
- ○
- ○
- ○

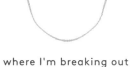

where I'm breaking out

EXTRA STEPS:

- ○ Exfoliation
- ○ Retinol
- ○ Face Mask
- ○
- ○

- ○
- ○
- ○
- ○
- ○

OTHER NOTES:

routine tracker

MORNING ROUTINE

TODAY MY SKIN FEELS:

TODAY I FEEL:

   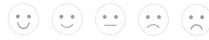

OTHER NOTES:

SKINCARE STEPS:

- ○ Cleanser
- ○ Toner
- ○ Spot Treatment
- ○ Serums
  - ○
  - ○
  - ○

- ○ Eye Cream
- ○ Moisturizer
- ○ Face Oil
- ○ Sunscreen
  - ○
  - ○
  - ○

where I'm breaking out

EXTRA STEPS:

- ○ Exfoliation
- ○ Face Mask
- ○ Face Massage
- ○
- ○

TOOLS I USED:

- ○ Gua Sha
- ○ Microcurrent Device
- ○ Jade Roller
- ○ Ice Roller
- ○

| 8oz | 8oz | 8oz | 8oz |

| 8oz | 8oz | 8oz | 8oz |

WATER INTAKE

184

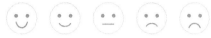
EVENING ROUTINE

TONIGHT MY SKIN FEELS:

TONIGHT I FEEL:

OTHER NOTES:

SKINCARE STEPS:

- ◯ Cleanser
- ◯ Toner
- ◯ Spot Treatment
- ◯ Serums
  - ◯
  - ◯
  - ◯

- ◯ Eye Cream
- ◯ Moisturizer
- ◯ Face Oil
- ◯
- ◯
- ◯
- ◯

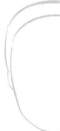

where I'm breaking out

EXTRA STEPS:

- ◯ Exfoliation
- ◯ Retinol
- ◯ Face Mask
- ◯
- ◯

- ◯
- ◯
- ◯
- ◯
- ◯

OTHER NOTES:

routine tracker

MORNING ROUTINE

TODAY MY SKIN FEELS:

TODAY I FEEL:

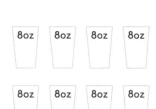

OTHER NOTES:

SKINCARE STEPS:

- ○ Cleanser
- ○ Toner
- ○ Spot Treatment
- ○ Serums
    - ○
    - ○
    - ○

- ○ Eye Cream
- ○ Moisturizer
- ○ Face Oil
- ○ Sunscreen
    - ○
    - ○
    - ○

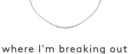

where I'm breaking out

EXTRA STEPS:

- ○ Exfoliation
- ○ Face Mask
- ○ Face Massage
- ○
- ○

TOOLS I USED:

- ○ Gua Sha
- ○ Microcurrent Device
- ○ Jade Roller
- ○ Ice Roller
- ○

8oz	8oz	8oz	8oz
8oz	8oz	8oz	8oz

WATER INTAKE

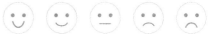

EVENING ROUTINE

TONIGHT MY SKIN FEELS:

TONIGHT I FEEL:

☺ ☺ 😐 🙁 🙁

OTHER NOTES:

SKINCARE STEPS:

- ○ Cleanser
- ○ Toner
- ○ Spot Treatment
- ○ Serums
  - ○
  - ○
  - ○

- ○ Eye Cream
- ○ Moisturizer
- ○ Face Oil
- ○
- ○
- ○
- ○

where I'm breaking out

EXTRA STEPS:

- ○ Exfoliation
- ○ Retinol
- ○ Face Mask
- ○
- ○

- ○
- ○
- ○
- ○
- ○

OTHER NOTES:

routine tracker

MORNING ROUTINE

TODAY MY SKIN FEELS:

TODAY I FEEL:

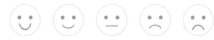

OTHER NOTES:

SKINCARE STEPS:

- ○ Cleanser
- ○ Toner
- ○ Spot Treatment
- ○ Serums
  - ○ _____
  - ○ _____
  - ○ _____

- ○ Eye Cream
- ○ Moisturizer
- ○ Face Oil
- ○ Sunscreen
  - ○ _____
  - ○ _____
  - ○ _____

where I'm breaking out

EXTRA STEPS:

- ○ Exfoliation
- ○ Face Mask
- ○ Face Massage
- ○ _____
- ○ _____

TOOLS I USED:

- ○ Gua Sha
- ○ Microcurrent Device
- ○ Jade Roller
- ○ Ice Roller
- ○ _____

8oz	8oz	8oz	8oz
8oz	8oz	8oz	8oz

WATER INTAKE

EVENING ROUTINE

TONIGHT MY SKIN FEELS:

TONIGHT I FEEL:

OTHER NOTES:

SKINCARE STEPS:

- ○ Cleanser
- ○ Toner
- ○ Spot Treatment
- ○ Serums
  - ○
  - ○
  - ○

- ○ Eye Cream
- ○ Moisturizer
- ○ Face Oil
- ○
- ○
- ○
- ○

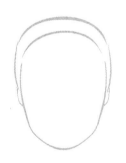

where I'm breaking out

EXTRA STEPS:

- ○ Exfoliation
- ○ Retinol
- ○ Face Mask
- ○
- ○

- ○
- ○
- ○
- ○
- ○

OTHER NOTES:

routine tracker

 date:

MORNING ROUTINE

TODAY MY SKIN FEELS:

TODAY I FEEL:

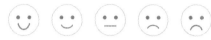

OTHER NOTES:

SKINCARE STEPS:

○ Cleanser   ○ Eye Cream
○ Toner   ○ Moisturizer
○ Spot Treatment   ○ Face Oil
○ Serums   ○ Sunscreen
　○   　○
　○   　○
　○   　○

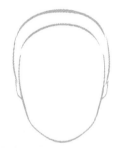

where I'm breaking out

EXTRA STEPS: TOOLS I USED:

○ Exfoliation   ○ Gua Sha
○ Face Mask   ○ Microcurrent Device
○ Face Massage   ○ Jade Roller
○   ○ Ice Roller
○   ○

8oz | 8oz | 8oz | 8oz

8oz | 8oz | 8oz | 8oz

WATER INTAKE

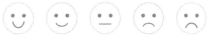

EVENING ROUTINE

TONIGHT MY SKIN FEELS:

TONIGHT I FEEL:

OTHER NOTES:

SKINCARE STEPS:

- ○ Cleanser
- ○ Toner
- ○ Spot Treatment
- ○ Serums
  - ○
  - ○
  - ○

- ○ Eye Cream
- ○ Moisturizer
- ○ Face Oil
- ○
- ○
- ○
- ○

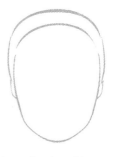

where I'm breaking out

EXTRA STEPS:

- ○ Exfoliation
- ○ Retinol
- ○ Face Mask
- ○
- ○

- ○
- ○
- ○
- ○
- ○

OTHER NOTES:

routine tracker

MORNING ROUTINE

TODAY MY SKIN FEELS:

TODAY I FEEL:

OTHER NOTES:

SKINCARE STEPS:

- ○ Cleanser
- ○ Toner
- ○ Spot Treatment
- ○ Serums
    - ○
    - ○
    - ○

- ○ Eye Cream
- ○ Moisturizer
- ○ Face Oil
- ○ Sunscreen
    - ○
    - ○
    - ○

where I'm breaking out

EXTRA STEPS:

- ○ Exfoliation
- ○ Face Mask
- ○ Face Massage
- ○
- ○

TOOLS I USED:

- ○ Gua Sha
- ○ Microcurrent Device
- ○ Jade Roller
- ○ Ice Roller
- ○

| 8oz | 8oz | 8oz | 8oz |
| 8oz | 8oz | 8oz | 8oz |

WATER INTAKE

EVENING ROUTINE

TONIGHT MY SKIN FEELS:

TONIGHT I FEEL:

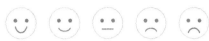

OTHER NOTES:

SKINCARE STEPS:

○ Cleanser   ○ Eye Cream
○ Toner   ○ Moisturizer
○ Spot Treatment   ○ Face Oil
○ Serums   ○
  ○   ○
  ○   ○
  ○   ○

where I'm breaking out

EXTRA STEPS:

○ Exfoliation   ○
○ Retinol   ○
○ Face Mask   ○
○   ○
○   ○

OTHER NOTES:

routine tracker

MORNING ROUTINE

TODAY MY SKIN FEELS:

TODAY I FEEL:

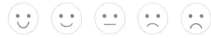

OTHER NOTES:

SKINCARE STEPS:

- ○ Cleanser
- ○ Toner
- ○ Spot Treatment
- ○ Serums
- ○ _____
- ○ _____
- ○ _____

- ○ Eye Cream
- ○ Moisturizer
- ○ Face Oil
- ○ Sunscreen
- ○ _____
- ○ _____
- ○ _____

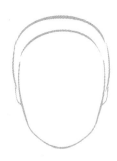

where I'm breaking out

EXTRA STEPS:

- ○ Exfoliation
- ○ Face Mask
- ○ Face Massage
- ○ _____
- ○ _____

TOOLS I USED:

- ○ Gua Sha
- ○ Microcurrent Device
- ○ Jade Roller
- ○ Ice Roller
- ○ _____

8oz	8oz	8oz	8oz
8oz	8oz	8oz	8oz

WATER INTAKE

EVENING ROUTINE

TONIGHT MY SKIN FEELS:

TONIGHT I FEEL:

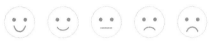

OTHER NOTES:

SKINCARE STEPS:

○ Cleanser   ○ Eye Cream
○ Toner   ○ Moisturizer
○ Spot Treatment ○ Face Oil
○ Serums   ○
    ○   ○
    ○   ○
    ○   ○

where I'm breaking out

EXTRA STEPS: OTHER NOTES:

○ Exfoliation   ○
○ Retinol   ○
○ Face Mask   ○
○   ○
○   ○

routine tracker

MORNING ROUTINE

TODAY MY SKIN FEELS:

TODAY I FEEL:

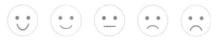

OTHER NOTES:

SKINCARE STEPS:

- ○ Cleanser
- ○ Toner
- ○ Spot Treatment
- ○ Serums
  - ○
  - ○
  - ○

- ○ Eye Cream
- ○ Moisturizer
- ○ Face Oil
- ○ Sunscreen
  - ○
  - ○
  - ○

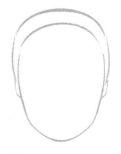

where I'm breaking out

EXTRA STEPS:

- ○ Exfoliation
- ○ Face Mask
- ○ Face Massage
- ○
- ○

TOOLS I USED:

- ○ Gua Sha
- ○ Microcurrent Device
- ○ Jade Roller
- ○ Ice Roller
- ○

8oz	8oz	8oz	8oz
8oz	8oz	8oz	8oz

WATER INTAKE

EVENING ROUTINE

TONIGHT MY SKIN FEELS:　　　　TONIGHT I FEEL:

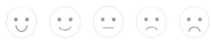

OTHER NOTES:

SKINCARE STEPS:

- ○ Cleanser
- ○ Toner
- ○ Spot Treatment
- ○ Serums
  - ○
  - ○
  - ○

- ○ Eye Cream
- ○ Moisturizer
- ○ Face Oil
- ○
- ○
- ○
- ○

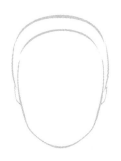

where I'm breaking out

EXTRA STEPS:　　　　　　　　　　OTHER NOTES:

- ○ Exfoliation
- ○ Retinol
- ○ Face Mask
- ○
- ○

- ○
- ○
- ○
- ○
- ○

routine tracker

 date:

MORNING ROUTINE

TODAY MY SKIN FEELS:

TODAY I FEEL:

OTHER NOTES:

SKINCARE STEPS:

- ○ Cleanser
- ○ Toner
- ○ Spot Treatment
- ○ Serums
  - ○
  - ○
  - ○

- ○ Eye Cream
- ○ Moisturizer
- ○ Face Oil
- ○ Sunscreen
  - ○
  - ○
  - ○

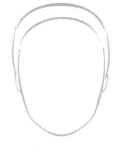

where I'm breaking out

EXTRA STEPS:

- ○ Exfoliation
- ○ Face Mask
- ○ Face Massage
- ○
- ○

TOOLS I USED:

- ○ Gua Sha
- ○ Microcurrent Device
- ○ Jade Roller
- ○ Ice Roller
- ○

| 8oz | 8oz | 8oz | 8oz |

| 8oz | 8oz | 8oz | 8oz |

WATER INTAKE

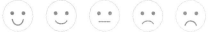
EVENING ROUTINE

TONIGHT MY SKIN FEELS:

TONIGHT I FEEL:

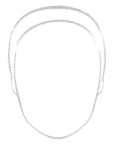

OTHER NOTES:

SKINCARE STEPS:

- ○ Cleanser
- ○ Toner
- ○ Spot Treatment
- ○ Serums
    - ○
    - ○
    - ○
- ○ Eye Cream
- ○ Moisturizer
- ○ Face Oil
- ○
- ○
- ○
- ○

where I'm breaking out

EXTRA STEPS:

- ○ Exfoliation
- ○ Retinol
- ○ Face Mask
- ○
- ○
- ○
- ○
- ○
- ○
- ○

OTHER NOTES:

routine tracker

MORNING ROUTINE

TODAY MY SKIN FEELS:

TODAY I FEEL:

OTHER NOTES:

SKINCARE STEPS:

- ○ Cleanser
- ○ Toner
- ○ Spot Treatment
- ○ Serums
  - ○
  - ○
  - ○

- ○ Eye Cream
- ○ Moisturizer
- ○ Face Oil
- ○ Sunscreen
  - ○
  - ○
  - ○

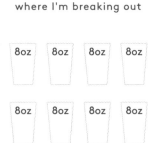

where I'm breaking out

EXTRA STEPS:

- ○ Exfoliation
- ○ Face Mask
- ○ Face Massage
- ○
- ○

TOOLS I USED:

- ○ Gua Sha
- ○ Microcurrent Device
- ○ Jade Roller
- ○ Ice Roller
- ○

8oz	8oz	8oz	8oz
8oz	8oz	8oz	8oz

WATER INTAKE

EVENING ROUTINE

TONIGHT MY SKIN FEELS:

TONIGHT I FEEL:

    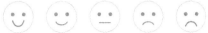

OTHER NOTES:

SKINCARE STEPS:

- ○ Cleanser
- ○ Toner
- ○ Spot Treatment
- ○ Serums
  - ○
  - ○
  - ○

- ○ Eye Cream
- ○ Moisturizer
- ○ Face Oil
- ○
- ○
- ○
- ○

where I'm breaking out

EXTRA STEPS:

- ○ Exfoliation
- ○ Retinol
- ○ Face Mask
- ○
- ○

- ○
- ○
- ○
- ○
- ○

OTHER NOTES:

routine tracker

MORNING ROUTINE

TODAY MY SKIN FEELS:

TODAY I FEEL:

OTHER NOTES:

SKINCARE STEPS:

- ○ Cleanser
- ○ Toner
- ○ Spot Treatment
- ○ Serums
  - ○
  - ○
  - ○

- ○ Eye Cream
- ○ Moisturizer
- ○ Face Oil
- ○ Sunscreen
  - ○
  - ○
  - ○

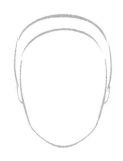

where I'm breaking out

EXTRA STEPS:

- ○ Exfoliation
- ○ Face Mask
- ○ Face Massage
- ○
- ○

TOOLS I USED:

- ○ Gua Sha
- ○ Microcurrent Device
- ○ Jade Roller
- ○ Ice Roller
- ○

WATER INTAKE

EVENING ROUTINE

TONIGHT MY SKIN FEELS:

TONIGHT I FEEL:

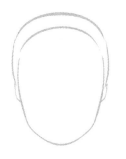

OTHER NOTES:

SKINCARE STEPS:

- ○ Cleanser
- ○ Toner
- ○ Spot Treatment
- ○ Serums
  - ○
  - ○
  - ○

- ○ Eye Cream
- ○ Moisturizer
- ○ Face Oil
- ○
- ○
- ○
- ○

where I'm breaking out

EXTRA STEPS:

- ○ Exfoliation
- ○ Retinol
- ○ Face Mask
- ○
- ○

- ○
- ○
- ○
- ○
- ○

OTHER NOTES:

routine tracker

MORNING ROUTINE

TODAY MY SKIN FEELS:

TODAY I FEEL:

OTHER NOTES:

SKINCARE STEPS:

- ○ Cleanser
- ○ Toner
- ○ Spot Treatment
- ○ Serums
  - ○
  - ○
  - ○

- ○ Eye Cream
- ○ Moisturizer
- ○ Face Oil
- ○ Sunscreen
  - ○
  - ○
  - ○

where I'm breaking out

EXTRA STEPS:

- ○ Exfoliation
- ○ Face Mask
- ○ Face Massage
- ○
- ○

TOOLS I USED:

- ○ Gua Sha
- ○ Microcurrent Device
- ○ Jade Roller
- ○ Ice Roller
- ○

8oz	8oz	8oz	8oz
8oz	8oz	8oz	8oz

WATER INTAKE

EVENING ROUTINE

TONIGHT MY SKIN FEELS:

TONIGHT I FEEL:

OTHER NOTES:

SKINCARE STEPS:

○ Cleanser   ○ Eye Cream
○ Toner   ○ Moisturizer
○ Spot Treatment   ○ Face Oil
○ Serums   ○
   ○   ○
   ○   ○
   ○   ○

where I'm breaking out

EXTRA STEPS: OTHER NOTES:

○ Exfoliation   ○
○ Retinol   ○
○ Face Mask   ○
○   ○
○   ○

routine tracker

MORNING ROUTINE

TODAY MY SKIN FEELS:

TODAY I FEEL:

OTHER NOTES:

SKINCARE STEPS:

○ Cleanser
○ Toner
○ Spot Treatment
○ Serums
　○
　○
　○

○ Eye Cream
○ Moisturizer
○ Face Oil
○ Sunscreen
○
○
○

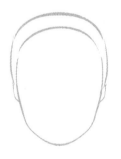

where I'm breaking out

EXTRA STEPS:

○ Exfoliation
○ Face Mask
○ Face Massage
○
○

TOOLS I USED:

○ Gua Sha
○ Microcurrent Device
○ Jade Roller
○ Ice Roller
○

8oz 8oz 8oz 8oz

8oz 8oz 8oz 8oz

WATER INTAKE

206

EVENING ROUTINE

TONIGHT MY SKIN FEELS: TONIGHT I FEEL:

  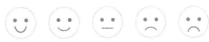

OTHER NOTES:

SKINCARE STEPS:

○ Cleanser   ○ Eye Cream
○ Toner   ○ Moisturizer
○ Spot Treatment   ○ Face Oil
○ Serums   ○
    ○   ○
    ○   ○
    ○   ○

where I'm breaking out

EXTRA STEPS: OTHER NOTES:

○ Exfoliation   ○
○ Retinol   ○
○ Face Mask   ○
○   ○
○   ○

routine tracker

MORNING ROUTINE

TODAY MY SKIN FEELS:

TODAY I FEEL:

OTHER NOTES:

SKINCARE STEPS:

- ○ Cleanser
- ○ Toner
- ○ Spot Treatment
- ○ Serums
  - ○
  - ○
  - ○
- ○ Eye Cream
- ○ Moisturizer
- ○ Face Oil
- ○ Sunscreen
  - ○
  - ○
  - ○

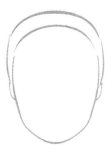

where I'm breaking out

EXTRA STEPS:

- ○ Exfoliation
- ○ Face Mask
- ○ Face Massage
- ○
- ○

TOOLS I USED:

- ○ Gua Sha
- ○ Microcurrent Device
- ○ Jade Roller
- ○ Ice Roller
- ○

| 8oz | 8oz | 8oz | 8oz |

| 8oz | 8oz | 8oz | 8oz |

WATER INTAKE

EVENING ROUTINE

TONIGHT MY SKIN FEELS:

TONIGHT I FEEL:

   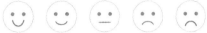

OTHER NOTES:

SKINCARE STEPS:

- ○ Cleanser
- ○ Toner
- ○ Spot Treatment
- ○ Serums
    - ○
    - ○
    - ○

- ○ Eye Cream
- ○ Moisturizer
- ○ Face Oil
- ○
- ○
- ○
- ○

where I'm breaking out

EXTRA STEPS:

- ○ Exfoliation
- ○ Retinol
- ○ Face Mask
- ○
- ○

- ○
- ○
- ○
- ○
- ○

OTHER NOTES:

routine tracker

MORNING ROUTINE

TODAY MY SKIN FEELS:

TODAY I FEEL:

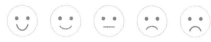

OTHER NOTES:

SKINCARE STEPS:

- ○ Cleanser
- ○ Toner
- ○ Spot Treatment
- ○ Serums
  - ○
  - ○
  - ○

- ○ Eye Cream
- ○ Moisturizer
- ○ Face Oil
- ○ Sunscreen
  - ○
  - ○
  - ○

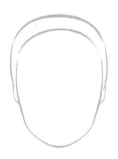

where I'm breaking out

EXTRA STEPS:

- ○ Exfoliation
- ○ Face Mask
- ○ Face Massage
- ○
- ○

TOOLS I USED:

- ○ Gua Sha
- ○ Microcurrent Device
- ○ Jade Roller
- ○ Ice Roller
- ○

8oz	8oz	8oz	8oz
8oz	8oz	8oz	8oz

WATER INTAKE

EVENING ROUTINE

TONIGHT MY SKIN FEELS:

TONIGHT I FEEL:

  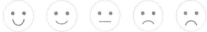

OTHER NOTES:

SKINCARE STEPS:

- ○ Cleanser
- ○ Toner
- ○ Spot Treatment
- ○ Serums
    - ○
    - ○
    - ○

- ○ Eye Cream
- ○ Moisturizer
- ○ Face Oil
- ○
- ○
- ○
- ○

where I'm breaking out

EXTRA STEPS:

- ○ Exfoliation
- ○ Retinol
- ○ Face Mask
- ○
- ○

- ○
- ○
- ○
- ○
- ○

OTHER NOTES:

routine tracker

 date:

MORNING ROUTINE

TODAY MY SKIN FEELS:

TODAY I FEEL:

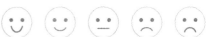

OTHER NOTES:

SKINCARE STEPS:

- ○ Cleanser
- ○ Toner
- ○ Spot Treatment
- ○ Serums
  - ○
  - ○
  - ○

- ○ Eye Cream
- ○ Moisturizer
- ○ Face Oil
- ○ Sunscreen
  - ○
  - ○
  - ○

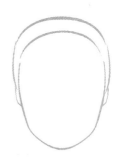

where I'm breaking out

EXTRA STEPS:

- ○ Exfoliation
- ○ Face Mask
- ○ Face Massage
- ○
- ○

TOOLS I USED:

- ○ Gua Sha
- ○ Microcurrent Device
- ○ Jade Roller
- ○ Ice Roller
- ○

8oz	8oz	8oz	8oz
8oz	8oz	8oz	8oz

WATER INTAKE

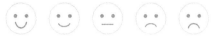
EVENING ROUTINE

TONIGHT MY SKIN FEELS:

TONIGHT I FEEL:

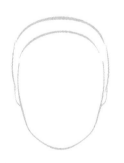

where I'm breaking out

OTHER NOTES:

SKINCARE STEPS:

- ○ Cleanser
- ○ Toner
- ○ Spot Treatment
- ○ Serums
    - ○
    - ○
    - ○

- ○ Eye Cream
- ○ Moisturizer
- ○ Face Oil
- ○
- ○
- ○
- ○

EXTRA STEPS:

- ○ Exfoliation
- ○ Retinol
- ○ Face Mask
- ○
- ○

- ○
- ○
- ○
- ○
- ○

OTHER NOTES:

routine tracker

MORNING ROUTINE

TODAY MY SKIN FEELS:

TODAY I FEEL:

OTHER NOTES:

SKINCARE STEPS:

- ○ Cleanser
- ○ Toner
- ○ Spot Treatment
- ○ Serums
  - ○
  - ○
  - ○

- ○ Eye Cream
- ○ Moisturizer
- ○ Face Oil
- ○ Sunscreen
  - ○
  - ○
  - ○

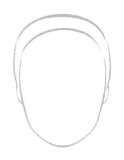

where I'm breaking out

EXTRA STEPS:

- ○ Exfoliation
- ○ Face Mask
- ○ Face Massage
- ○
- ○

TOOLS I USED:

- ○ Gua Sha
- ○ Microcurrent Device
- ○ Jade Roller
- ○ Ice Roller
- ○

| 8oz | 8oz | 8oz | 8oz |
| 8oz | 8oz | 8oz | 8oz |

WATER INTAKE

EVENING ROUTINE

TONIGHT MY SKIN FEELS:

TONIGHT I FEEL:

   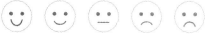

OTHER NOTES:

SKINCARE STEPS:

- ○ Cleanser
- ○ Toner
- ○ Spot Treatment
- ○ Serums
  - ○
  - ○
  - ○

- ○ Eye Cream
- ○ Moisturizer
- ○ Face Oil
- ○
- ○
- ○
- ○

where I'm breaking out

EXTRA STEPS:

- ○ Exfoliation
- ○ Retinol
- ○ Face Mask
- ○
- ○

- ○
- ○
- ○
- ○
- ○

OTHER NOTES:

routine tracker

MORNING ROUTINE

TODAY MY SKIN FEELS:

TODAY I FEEL:

    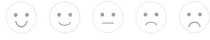

OTHER NOTES:

SKINCARE STEPS:

- ○ Cleanser
- ○ Toner
- ○ Spot Treatment
- ○ Serums
  - ○
  - ○
  - ○

- ○ Eye Cream
- ○ Moisturizer
- ○ Face Oil
- ○ Sunscreen
  - ○
  - ○
  - ○

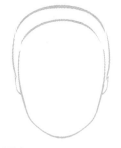

where I'm breaking out

EXTRA STEPS:

- ○ Exfoliation
- ○ Face Mask
- ○ Face Massage
- ○
- ○

TOOLS I USED:

- ○ Gua Sha
- ○ Microcurrent Device
- ○ Jade Roller
- ○ Ice Roller
- ○

| 8oz | 8oz | 8oz | 8oz |
| 8oz | 8oz | 8oz | 8oz |

WATER INTAKE

EVENING ROUTINE

TONIGHT MY SKIN FEELS:

TONIGHT I FEEL:

OTHER NOTES:

SKINCARE STEPS:

- ○ Cleanser
- ○ Toner
- ○ Spot Treatment
- ○ Serums
  - ○
  - ○
  - ○

- ○ Eye Cream
- ○ Moisturizer
- ○ Face Oil
- ○
- ○
- ○
- ○

where I'm breaking out

EXTRA STEPS:

- ○ Exfoliation
- ○ Retinol
- ○ Face Mask
- ○
- ○

- ○
- ○
- ○
- ○
- ○

OTHER NOTES:

routine tracker

MORNING ROUTINE

TODAY MY SKIN FEELS:

TODAY I FEEL:

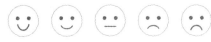

OTHER NOTES:

SKINCARE STEPS:

- ○ Cleanser
- ○ Toner
- ○ Spot Treatment
- ○ Serums
  - ○
  - ○
  - ○

- ○ Eye Cream
- ○ Moisturizer
- ○ Face Oil
- ○ Sunscreen
  - ○
  - ○
  - ○

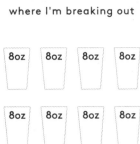

where I'm breaking out

EXTRA STEPS:

- ○ Exfoliation
- ○ Face Mask
- ○ Face Massage
- ○
- ○

TOOLS I USED:

- ○ Gua Sha
- ○ Microcurrent Device
- ○ Jade Roller
- ○ Ice Roller
- ○

8oz	8oz	8oz	8oz
8oz	8oz	8oz	8oz

WATER INTAKE

EVENING ROUTINE

TONIGHT MY SKIN FEELS:

TONIGHT I FEEL:

OTHER NOTES:

SKINCARE STEPS:

○ Cleanser   ○ Eye Cream
○ Toner   ○ Moisturizer
○ Spot Treatment ○ Face Oil
○ Serums   ○
    ○   ○
    ○   ○
    ○   ○

where I'm breaking out

EXTRA STEPS:

OTHER NOTES:

○ Exfoliation   ○
○ Retinol   ○
○ Face Mask   ○
○   ○
○   ○

219

routine tracker

MORNING ROUTINE

TODAY MY SKIN FEELS:

TODAY I FEEL:

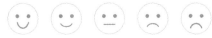

OTHER NOTES:

SKINCARE STEPS:

- ◯ Cleanser
- ◯ Toner
- ◯ Spot Treatment
- ◯ Serums
    - ◯
    - ◯
    - ◯

- ◯ Eye Cream
- ◯ Moisturizer
- ◯ Face Oil
- ◯ Sunscreen
    - ◯
    - ◯
    - ◯

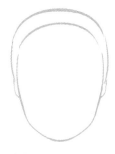

where I'm breaking out

EXTRA STEPS:

- ◯ Exfoliation
- ◯ Face Mask
- ◯ Face Massage
- ◯
- ◯

TOOLS I USED:

- ◯ Gua Sha
- ◯ Microcurrent Device
- ◯ Jade Roller
- ◯ Ice Roller
- ◯

8oz	8oz	8oz	8oz
8oz	8oz	8oz	8oz

WATER INTAKE

EVENING ROUTINE

TONIGHT MY SKIN FEELS:

TONIGHT I FEEL:

OTHER NOTES:

SKINCARE STEPS:

○ Cleanser   ○ Eye Cream
○ Toner   ○ Moisturizer
○ Spot Treatment   ○ Face Oil
○ Serums   ○
    ○   ○
    ○   ○
    ○   ○

where I'm breaking out

EXTRA STEPS:

OTHER NOTES:

○ Exfoliation   ○
○ Retinol   ○
○ Face Mask   ○
○   ○
○   ○

Additional Resources

Looking for more information on skin care?
Here are some great resources to help you continue on your journey!

WEBSITES

American Academy of Dermatology at aad.org/public
Information vetted by top dermatologists in the country.

Cleveland Clinic at my.clevelandclinic.org
A comprehensive medical resource that covers topics relating to skin care.

The Derm Review at thedermreview.com
Product reviews straight from dermatologists.

Dermstore at dermstore.com
Not only a great place to purchase skincare products but also a useful source of medically backed information.

EWG's Skin Deep at ewg.org/skindeep
The Environmental Working Group's database on what, exactly, is in your products.

Good Housekeeping at goodhousekeeping.com
The gold standard in product testing and reviews for nearly one hundred and fifty years.

Mayo Clinic at mayoclinic.org
Another helpful medically backed resource, especially regarding skin disorders.

Reddit at reddit.com
There is a bustling skincare community on Reddit, especially on subreddits like r/skincareaddiction.

The Skin Cancer Foundation at skincancer.org
A go-to resource for all things skin health.

Total Beauty at totalbeauty.com
Another excellent site for in-depth reviews and tips. It provides nitty-gritty breakdowns on whether a product is worth it or not, as well as roundups of new products.

BOOKS

Black Skin: The Definitive Skincare Guide by Dija Ayodele
Skin with more melanin can sometimes require a different set of tips. This book breaks them down.

Ayodele, Dija. *Black Skin: The Definitive Skincare Guide* (Huntington, WV: HQ, 2022).

Glow from Within by Joanna Vargas
One of the top aestheticians in the industry shares her secrets to glowing skin.

Vargas, Joanna. *Glow from Within* (New York: Harper Wave, 2020).

Let's Face It by Rio Viera-Newton
Viera-Newton is the skincare guru of *New York* magazine, and in this book, she helps readers put together a routine that works for them.

Viera-Newton, Rio. *Let's Face It* (Boston: Little, Brown, 2021).

The Little Book of Skin Care by Charlotte Cho
The founder of Korean beauty brand Soko Glam helps readers adopt a skin-first approach to beauty.

Cho, Charlotte. *The Little Book of Skin Care* (New York: William Morrow, 2015).

Palette: The Beauty Bible for Women of Color by Funmi Fetto
A guide to skincare and beauty essentials for Black skin from a veteran beauty editor.

Fetto, Funmi. *Palette: The Beauty Bible for Women of Color* (London: Quercus, 2020).

Skincare: The New Edit by Caroline Hirons
The original guide to skin care, this new edition dives into more complex topics, including puberty and endometriosis and how they affect the skin.

Hirons, Caroline. *Skincare: The New Edit* (Huntington, WV: HQ, 2022).

The Skincare Bible: Your No-Nonsense Guide to Great Skin by Anjali Mahto
An in-depth guide to ingredients, skin function, and other questions around skin care from a dermatologist.

Mahto, Anjali. *The Skincare Bible: Your No-Nonsense Guide to Great Skin* (New York: Penguin Life, 2018).

Skincare Decoded by Victoria Fu and Gloria Lu
Written by skincare chemists, this book deciphers the most complicated skincare terms and questions.

Fu, Victoria, and Gloria Lu. *Skincare Decoded* (San Rafael, CA: Weldon Owen, 2021).

Your Best Skin: The Science of Skincare by Hannah English
An unbiased, science-first resource compiled by a veteran beauty journalist.

English, Hannah. *Your Best Skin: The Science of Skincare* (San Francisco: Hardie Grant, 2022).

Your Future Face: The Customized Plan to Look Younger at Any Age by Dennis Gross
One of the original skincare gurus, Dr. Gross guides readers through a holistic approach to skin care, including products, diet, and more.

Gross, Dennis. *Your Future Face: The Customized Plan to Look Younger at Any Age* (New York: Viking, 2004).

PODCASTS

Breaking Beauty at breakingbeautypodcast.com
Two longtime beauty editors cut through the beauty BS and deliver all the information you need to take control of your routine.

Fat Mascara at fatmascara.com
One of the most popular beauty podcasts out there; veteran beauty editors discuss tips, trends, and more with a rotating cast of professionals.

Gloss Angeles at glossangelespod.com/episodes-blog
Two beauty pros with years of experience break down the latest in beauty and skincare trends through a pop culture lens.

Glowing Up at podcasts.apple.com/us/podcast/glowing-up/id1255335865
Two beauty obsessives discuss the products they're testing and whether they're worth the hype.

The Science of Beauty at podcasts.apple.com/us/podcast/allure-the-science-of-beauty/id1531535720
A super granular look at the specifics of beauty, including episodes dedicated to specific ingredients.

SKINCARE TELEMEDICINE

Agency at withagency.com
While this digital derm only deals in custom retinol products, it customizes your experience with the help of photos that you upload on a regular schedule.

Apostrophe at apostrophe.com
This fully online dermatologist connects you with doctors via video app and provides both topical and oral medications.

Curology at curology.com
A full-service digital dermatologist that provides personalized medication on a subscription basis to help treat fine lines and acne.

About the Author

Maria Del Russo is a writer, editor, and branded content consultant specializing in women's issues, relationships, wellness, and beauty. She has written for *Cosmopolitan*, *Refinery29*, *Elle*, *Playboy*, *InStyle*, and many other digital and print publications. She also writes a weekly newsletter, *Sunday Sauce*, in which she cooks her way through her family's Italian-American recipes. Maria lives in Brooklyn with her partner, Ben, and their dog, Edie. She is the author of *Daily Skincare Journal* and *Simple Acts of Love*.